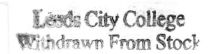

D0246374

Adolescent Health

Series Editor: Cara Acred

Volume 252

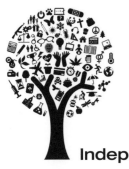

Independence Educational Publishers

First published by Independence Educational Publishers

The Studio, High Green

Great Shelford

Cambridge CB22 5EG

England

© Independence 2013

Photocopy licence

The material in this book is protected by copyright. However, the
purchaser is free to make multiple copies of particular articles for instructional
purposes for immediate use within the purchasing institution.
Making copies of the entire book is not permitted.

British Library Cataloguing in Publication Data

Adolescent health. -- (Issues ; 252)

1. Teenagers--Health and hygiene. 2. Health behaviour in
adolescence.

I. Series II. Acred, Cara editor of compilation.

613'.0433-dc23

ISBN-13: 9781861686589

Printed in Great Britain
MWL Print Group Ltd

Contents

Introduction

Adolescent Health is Volume 252 in the *ISSUES* series. The aim of the series is to offer current, diverse information about important issues in our world, from a UK perspective.

ABOUT ADOLESCENT HEALTH

Teenagers today are taking fewer illegal drugs and drinking less alcohol. This is, undoubtedly, good news. However, rates of sexually transmitted diseases among young people are increasing and a dangerous new trend sees students turning to 'smart' drugs to boost exam performance. Worryingly, diagnoses of long-term conditions such as diabetes, epilepsy and asthma are also on the rise, as is teenage obesity. This book explores the different issues involved in adolescent health, considering teenagers' views on their health experiences and looking at areas such as teen depression, exam stress, lack of sleep and 'risky' behaviour.

OUR SOURCES

Titles in the *ISSUES* series are designed to function as educational resource books, providing a balanced overview of a specific subject.

The information in our books is comprised of facts, articles and opinions from many different sources, including:

⇨ Newspaper reports and opinion pieces

⇨ Website factsheets

⇨ Magazine and journal articles

⇨ Statistics and surveys

⇨ Government reports

⇨ Literature from special interest groups

A NOTE ON CRITICAL EVALUATION

Because the information reprinted here is from a number of different sources, readers should bear in mind the origin of the text and whether the source is likely to have a particular bias when presenting information (or when conducting their research). It is hoped that, as you read about the many aspects of the issues explored in this book, you will critically evaluate the information presented.

It is important that you decide whether you are being presented with facts or opinions. Does the writer give a biased or unbiased report? If an opinion is being expressed, do you agree with the writer? Is there potential bias to the 'facts' or statistics behind an article?

ASSIGNMENTS

In the back of this book, you will find a selection of assignments designed to help you engage with the articles you have been reading and to explore your own opinions. Some tasks will take longer than others and there is a mixture of design, writing and research based activities that you can complete alone or in a group.

FURTHER RESEARCH

At the end of each article we have listed its source and a website that you can visit if you would like to conduct your own research. Please remember to critically evaluate any sources that you consult and consider whether the information you are viewing is accurate and unbiased.

Useful weblinks

www.anxietyuk.org.uk

www.ayph.org.uk

www.bupa.co.uk

www.childline.org.uk

www.mentalhealth.org.uk

www.ncb.org.uk

www.youngminds.org.uk

Adolescent health in the UK today

Update 2012.

Dr Ann Hagell, Co-Development Manager, AYPH, and Dr John Coleman OBE, Senior Research Fellow, University of Oxford, AYPH Chair

Key trends in adolescent health

There are two general views of adolescent health. On one hand, adolescence can be regarded as a time of general good health and physical fitness. This is not a life period dominated by the big threats of older age; heart problems, cancer and lung disease for example. In addition, medical advances have helped in the management of chronic conditions such as asthma and childhood diabetes. However, the second view is that there is, in fact, much to be worried about; if asked about health in this age group many professionals would mention widespread use of alcohol, rising levels of obesity and worrying rates of sexually transmitted infections. As researchers have pointed out, there have been significant improvements in overall health outcomes in the last few decades among all age groups apart from adolescence.[1] For example, mortality rates amongst young people aged 15-19 and 20-24 have risen above rates for those in the one to four age group, a reversal of historical mortality trends.

Overall, taking both perspectives into account, a careful look at the trends for young people's health shows that the picture is much more nuanced than we might assume, with areas which show little change, others where there have indeed been significant improvements, and yet others where things have got worse.

Looking first at the improvements, it is encouraging to recognise that the rate of teenage conceptions has shown a significant reduction over the last ten years, and that trend has continued since our last update in 2011. Previously, we noted that conception rates for under-16s and under-18s had fallen in England and Wales since the introduction of the national Teenage Pregnancy Strategy in 1998. The most recent statistics in 2010 showed the trend continuing. The under-18 conception rate had fallen again, to 35.5 per 1,000 girls aged 15-17, down from 47.1 in 1998, and the lowest rate for decades.[2]

Another area of significant improvement relates to suicide rates among 15- to 24-year-old young men. Rates here have fallen over the last ten years from 16.5 per 100,000 in 2000, to 10.5 per 100,000 in the latest statistics from 2009.[3] The equivalent statistics for young women were 4.4 in 2000, down to three in 2009. This means the actual number of recorded suicides and undetermined deaths in the UK fell by nearly one quarter from 2000 to 2009 (from 742 to 568), with young men accounting for nearly 80% of these deaths. There has, however, been little change in rates of self-harm, although

this is an area where getting good statistics is notoriously difficult. We should also note considerable regional variation in these figures; in 2009, suicide rates among young adult males were very much higher in Northern Ireland (25.5 per 100,000) and Scotland (20.9) than in Wales (12.2) and England (8.7).

Turning to substance use, here again many of the trends continue to go in the right direction, as can be seen from evidence gained from studies carried out by the NHS Information Centre, the Health Behaviour in School-aged Children studies, the Department of Health funded SDDU studies, and the European ESPAD.[4] Overall, the extent of substance misuse has reduced substantially among 13- and 15-year-olds in England and Scotland since 2002. In England, the proportion of 15-year-old boys who reported having tried illegal drugs reduced from 39% to 27% between 2002 and 2010. Among the same group in Scotland, the proportion reduced from 35% to 21%. There have always been gender differences in drug use; at age 13, for example, the proportions of young people taking drugs are quite similar among girls and boys, but by the age of 15, higher proportions of boys report having taken illegal drugs. There are also gender differences in the country comparisons: at age 15, the extent of drug use among

1 Lancet Editorial (2012) *Putting adolescents at the centre of health and development.* The Lancet, 379, p1561

2 Gale E (2011) *Diabetes in the UK: time for a reality check?* Diabetic Medicine, 27, 973-976

3 Dalding, J (2000) *Young people into 2000.* Schools Health Education Unit. Exeter University. Exeter.

4 Madge N, Flood S, Laws S and Loeb D (2005) *Children and young people's views on health and health services a review of the evidence.* London. National Children's Bureau

young females is 50% higher in England than in the rest of Great Britain. Of illegal drugs, cannabis is the most commonly used, with recent statistics suggesting that 21% of 15-year-olds in England and 17% in Scotland having tried it in the last year; again, these figures represent an improvement over recent years. There is good news about cigarette smoking as well. Among 16- to 19-year-olds in Britain over a 25-year period, the proportion who smokes has fallen from a third to a fifth, but we remain concerned about smoking by young women, who smoke more than young men. Use of alcohol is more widespread and the trends are more complicated; we return to these below.

In terms of mental health, there is conflicting evidence, and it is hard to pin down recent trends. Taking the long-term view, evidence from the big British birth cohort studies shows increasing rates of mental health symptoms (particularly anxiety, depression and conduct disorder) among 16-year-olds between the mid-1970s and the late 1990s.[5] Levels of mental health problems among this age group appear higher now than they did 30 years ago. However, the trends since 2000 are less clear. Where studies of psychiatric morbidity are concerned, little change has been discerned between the years 1999 and 2004, with rates for 11-15 year-olds staying at around 10%.[6,7] There have been no new data on this since our last update, but the data on reductions in suicide rates are encouraging as they will be related to other mental health trends.

This relatively positive picture has to be balanced against some trends which give rise to significant concerns. As far as alcohol use is concerned, the picture is mixed. The proportion of young people who drink alcohol has reduced substantially in the last decade across Great Britain – from approaching 50% of 15-year-olds in England in 2002 to around 30% today.[8] The levels are slightly higher in Wales and Scotland. However, among those who do drink, the average amount of alcohol they consume in a week has increased since the mid-1990s, and in England, the average amount consumed in the last week by 11-13 year olds who drink has trebled since 1994, from 4.1 to 12.1 units today. Among 15-year-olds, average consumption levels doubled over the same period, from 6.4 to 12.9 units (note, however, that measurement of units has changed, which may have contributed).[9]

Rising rates of sexually transmitted infections have also been of major concern, with chlamydia and herpes and genital warts showing particularly marked changes among young people. New diagnoses of chlamydia are the most significant, having increased by 25% over the past ten years. However, numbers may have peaked in 2008 and appear to have fallen back substantially over the past two years from a high of 28,612 in 2008 to 21,655 in 2010, a reduction of 24% in just two years. Screening patterns may have contributed, and these trends need to be verified as reflecting underlying disease status, not policy and practice shifts. Interestingly, while the same pattern is evident in new cases of genital warts (rise to 2008 then falling since), a different pattern is seen with new cases of herpes, where numbers are continuing to rise.

In addition to these trends, two other aspects of adolescent health give cause for anxiety. The first of these has to do with obesity, as around one third of young people aged 11–15 are overweight, and around one in six are obese (18% in England, 14% in Scotland). However, the proportions falling into these categories have fluctuated over the last 15 years. Indeed, although the levels in England appear to have reduced slightly since 2003/4, they are not significantly different today than proportions recorded in the late 1990s. The relation between exercise and weight is not clear-cut, and there will be many factors apart from physical activity that influence weight. That said, the recommended physical activity level for children in their mid-teens is at least 60 minutes of moderate-to-vigorous activity every day. Revised questions in the 2008 Health Survey for England led to much lower (and, it is believed, more accurate) levels of self-reported physical activity being recorded than previously. These latest data suggest that the proportion of young people aged 11-15 who meet the minimum requirement may be less than one quarter.

The final concern giving anxiety is the increase in long-term conditions such as epilepsy, asthma and diabetes. The number of hospital admissions for adolescents with long-term conditions has increased substantially since 2002/3. In 2009/10, nearly 22,600 11-19 year olds with diabetes, asthma or epilepsy were admitted to hospital, and increase of 26% since 2002/3. The highest increases (31%) were recorded for adolescents with diabetes.

⇨ The above information is reprinted with kind permission from the Association for Young People's Health. Please visit www.ayph.org.uk for further information.

© 2012 Association for Young People's Health

5 MacPherson A (2005) *ABC of adolescence: Adolescents in primary care*. British Medical Journal, 330, 465-467

6 Hargreaves D and Viner R (2011) *Children's and young people's experience of the National Health Service in England: a review of national surveys 2001-2011*. Archives of Disease in Childhood. (Online first: doi:10.1136/archdischild-2011-300603)

7 Coleman J, Brooks F and Treadgold P (2011) *Key Data on Adolescence, 2011*. London: Association for Young People's Health

8 Viner RM, Coffey C, Mathers C et al (2011) *50 year mortality trends in children and young people: a study of 50 low-income, middle-income and high-income countries*. Lancet, 377, 1162-74

9 Viner R and Barker M (2005) *Young People's health: the need for action*. British Medical Journal 330, 901-3

Ten reasons for investing in young people's health

There are 7.6 million young people aged ten to 19 in the UK, making up 12% of the population. AYPH believes it is important to invest in their health, because:

1. Adolescence is a critical time for health

This age marks the beginning of risk-taking behaviour, the start of a sexual life, the first manifestation of many serious long-term conditions, and a time when life-long health behaviours are set in place.

2. Adolescent health is not improving enough

The Lancet recently reported higher rates of mortality in this age group than previously and no significant health improvements compared to other age groups. Teen cancer is the leading cause of non-accidental death in young people in the UK. Over 2,500 young people aged 13-24 years are diagnosed each year.

3. Young people are not getting the health services or information they require

They are regular users of primary care, but report a lack of satisfaction with communication and understanding of confidentiality.

4. Good sexual health services, in particular, are critical

In 2011, 2.1 million chlamydia tests were carried out in England among young adults (15 to 24 years), with over 147,000 diagnoses made. But the chlamydia diagnosis rate dropped by four per cent from 2010-11. This trend must be continued to meet the Public Health Outcomes Framework recommendation.

5. Teenage pregnancy reduction must continue

Under-18 conception rates for 2010 were the lowest in England since 1969, achieved by intense work at local level. That effort must continue or rates will start to rise again.

6. Ignoring chronic adolescent disease costs money

This leads to more emergency admissions. Diabetes, asthma and epilepsy in this age group resulted in 21,600 hospitalisations in England in 2009-10.

7. Effects of poor youth health care can last a lifetime

One third of those aged 11-15 in the UK are overweight, one in six obese. Less than half meet minimum exercise requirements and one fifth of 16- to 19-year-olds smoke. These behaviours have long-term health costs unless they are tackled.

8. Investing in adolescent health has benefits across the spectrum

29% of young people in England aged 15 have experimented with illegal drugs at some point and 28% are drinking regularly, which impacts on crime levels, accidents and A&E admissions.

9. Health inequalities become established

Poverty and health are intertwined from birth. Adolescence represents a final chance to intervene, before the next generation arrives.

10. Important new research has brought new insights

For example, about the ongoing development of the brain, setting a new context for how we think about adolescent health. New data recently confirmed that smoking cannabis before 18 can result in long-term damage to the teen brain.

⇨ The above information is reprinted with kind permission from the Association for Young People's Health. Please visit www.ayph.org.uk for further information.

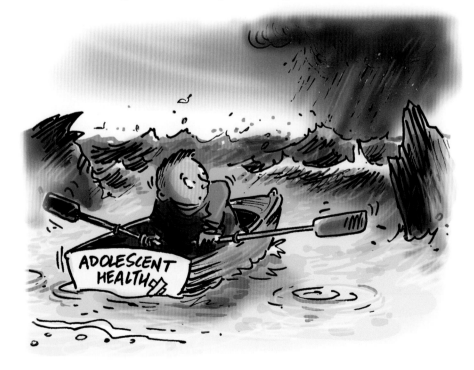

Teenagers' views on their health and local health services

Young people are major users of healthcare services

⇨ Around ten percent of consultations in GP surgeries are for children aged 14 and under.[1]

⇨ A school-age child will see their GP on average between two and three times per year.[2]

⇨ Children account for around 40 per cent of the workload of a typical GP.[2]

Government is currently making significant changes to the way NHS and public health services are planned and delivered, with a greater role for GPs and local authorities. Central to the reforms is government's ambition to give patients and the public a greater say in decisions about health services and their own care. If these reforms are to work for young people in England, it is imperative that their views and opinions are

1 NHS Information Centre (2008a) Research report on trends in consultation rates in general practices 1995-2008

2 Kennedy Review (2010) Getting it right for children and young people: overcoming cultural barriers in the NHS so as to meet their needs

taken into consideration as changes are implemented and embedded. During October to December 2011 the National Children's Bureau, assisted by b-live Foundation, undertook an online survey of young people aged 11 to 19 to find out their views on their own health and health services. The survey was hosted on the b-live website and was open to b-live members and other young people, including Young NCB members. Overall, 263 young people completed the questionnaire. While the sample was self-selecting and therefore not necessarily representative of England's young people, responses were received from young people across a range of ages, ethnic backgrounds and experiences.

How healthy are young people?

The young people we consulted were asked a series of questions to get a sense of their current lifestyle and how healthy they felt.

Key findings

⇨ The majority (86 per cent) felt confident that their health was good or very good while only two respondents thought it was bad or very bad.

⇨ The majority had eaten breakfast, eaten fruit and taken time to relax the day before completing the survey.

⇨ However, a substantial minority (almost a quarter) said they had eaten fast food (such as chips, burgers and kebabs) the previous day, and even more suggested that they had not exercised for 30 minutes or more.

⇨ Over half of our respondents had eight or more hours sleep the night prior to answering our survey. However, just over one in ten had five hours or less.

⇨ The majority (86 per cent) of respondents said that they had felt stressed due to a number of different things in the week prior to answering the survey. By far, the most common causes of stress identified by the young people was school work and exams, which had made six out of ten feel stressed in the week previous to completing the survey. Other significant causes of stress, each experienced by around one third of respondents in the last week, were: their future career, their physical appearance, friends, and family relationships. Money worries had made a quarter of respondents feel stressed.

Health information, advice and support

Young people were asked to tell us about where they got health advice and information, who they turned to for support and what sort of health information they need.

Key findings

⇨ Parents are an important source of health advice for the young

Health behaviours of young people aged 11 to 19 years old*

* Overall, 263 young people were consulted. For this question, young people were asked to identify which health behaviours they carried out the previous day.

Source: Teenagers' views on their health and local health services, 2012. National Children's Bureau.

people we consulted. They were the most commonly cited source of health information and the people whose advice the young people said they would most pay attention to. Parents were also the most popular source of support if the young people were worried about their health.

⇨ Some young people felt uncomfortable about visiting their GP. Under half of respondents said they got most of their health information from a health clinic, and just under half said they would talk to their GP if they were worried about their health. However, while the majority said they were very or quite comfortable visiting their GP, over a quarter said they were not. The most common causes of feeling uncomfortable while visiting their GP were: feeling embarrassed, finding it hard to explain their problem, feeling like they were being judged, and not understanding what the doctor was saying to them.

⇨ Friends were more a source of support about health issues than a source of health information. Only a quarter of respondents cited friends as a source of health information, and less than one in ten would rely most on the health advice of a friend. However, peer groups were identified as a source of support for many, with half saying they would turn to a friend if they were worried about their health.

⇨ While there is a popular perception that teenagers are heavily influenced by celebrities and personalities, only four per cent of our respondents said that they would pay attention to the health advice or example set by an actor, musician, sports personality or TV star.

⇨ Over half of the young people felt they needed more information about reducing stress and just under half wanted more information

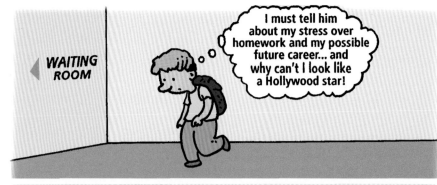

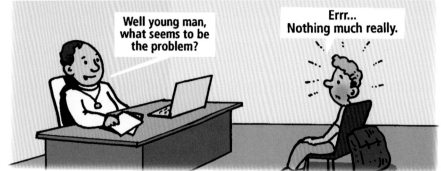

about places they could get help locally.

Conclusion and recommendations

Findings from our survey about young people's sources of health information echo messages from other studies of young people's views, for example on careers choices,[3] which see young people turning to their parents first for advice on a range of issues. However, it is important to bear in mind that parents will need support and advice to have the knowledge and understanding to inform their children's health management. As part of government's approach to improving the health of our population, there needs to be a clear strategy which targets parents and carers as co-educators of children and young people on health issues.

While, for the young people we consulted, GPs and health professionals were another important source of health information, they also expressed some reservations. Over a quarter said they did not feel comfortable visiting their doctor – some feel embarrassed or judged or find it hard to explain their health

problems. Health Education England, which will be established in 2012 to provide national leadership on health workforce development should ensure all health practitioners are able to effectively communicate with and support young people in looking after their own health and making decisions about healthcare. Local health services should also involve young people themselves in evaluating the quality of services and making recommendations for improvement, as recommended in the Government's *Positive for Youth* policy statement.[4]

Only a small minority of respondents to our survey (14 per cent) said they had not felt stressed in the previous week. The most commonly cited sources of stress were school work or exams, concerns about their future career, and their physical appearance. With recent reports indicating that unemployment for 16- to 26-year-olds is now over one million,[5]

3 NCB/BYC (2009) Young people's views on finding out about jobs and careers. NCB

4 HM Government (2011) Positive for Youth: new approach to cross-government policy for young people aged 13 to 19. Participation Work's The Young Inspectors Package offers tailored suites of resources and training along with dedicated consultancy time to enable organisations to meaningfully involve young people in evaluating their services www.participationworks.org.uk/topics/young-inspectors

5 For example Guardian, 16 November 2011, Youth unemployment hits 1 million

we cannot be surprised that many young people are worried about their future prospects. Furthermore, with a challenging economic environment, we may see this increase as a source of stress and worry for young people. It is also worth noting that the survey was conducted in the autumn so not even at peak exam time, when we may expect exam stress to be even greater than usual. Almost a quarter of the respondents rated money worries as a stress inducer, which may indicate a need for more and better quality financial literacy support, something members of Young NCB have been calling for through their Get Money Savvy campaign.[6]

With one in ten five- to 16-year-olds in the UK having a clinically diagnosable mental health

6   www.facebook.com/getmoneysavvy

problem[7], local and national policy must address the sources of stress for this age group, which could, result in more serious problems down the line. It is vital that:

⇨   the Youth Contract, the Government's programme for securing jobs, apprenticeships and work experience for young people, delivers real opportunities for young people, and young people understand how they can benefit from these sorts of programmes

⇨   those planning and delivering health services for young people work with other services in the area (such as schools and youth services) to address the impact of these concerns on young people's sense of well-being.

The second most popular issue on which the young people wanted

7   Office for National Statistics data for 2004. Green, H., McGinnity, A., Meltzer, T Ford, and R Goodman (2004) Mental health in children and young people in Great Britain. Basingstoke: Palgrave MacMillan

information was where to get help locally. The Department of Health must ensure that young people are a central part of the development and implementation of its forthcoming information strategy, ensuring young people have access to appropriate information about health concerns and the availability and quality of local services.

February 2012

⇨   National Children's Bureau (2012) *Teenagers' views on their health and local health services*. London: National Children's Bureau.

⇨   Please visit www.ncb.org.uk for further information.

© *National Children's Bureau 2013*

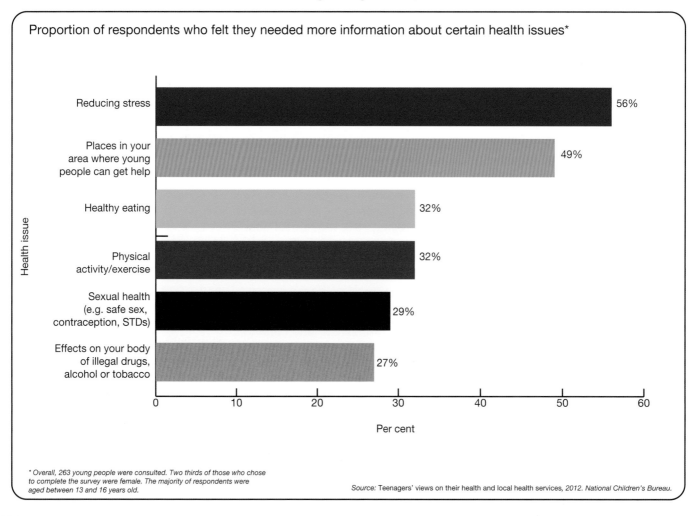

Proportion of respondents who felt they needed more information about certain health issues*

Health issue

Reducing stress — 56%
Places in your area where young people can get help — 49%
Healthy eating — 32%
Physical activity/exercise — 32%
Sexual health (e.g. safe sex, contraception, STDs) — 29%
Effects on your body of illegal drugs, alcohol or tobacco — 27%

Per cent

* Overall, 263 young people were consulted. Two thirds of those who chose to complete the survey were female. The majority of respondents were aged between 13 and 16 years old.

Source: Teenagers' views on their health and local health services, 2012. National Children's Bureau.

Long-term conditions

AYPH research summary.

Introduction

This Research Update provides an overview of long-term conditions affecting adolescents. It complements an earlier update on Disability that we produced last April and covers a selection of recent reports and research, as well as the latest data and policy guidance.

Long-term conditions that cannot be cured are a highly significant concern for growing numbers of young people and their families. They also present very major challenges for health service professionals and others involved in providing age-appropriate treatment, care and support.

Results for England from the latest HBSC[1] study found that 15% of all school students aged 11-15 report having been diagnosed with a long-term illness, disability or medical condition. This increasing prevalence of long-term conditions has led to greater attention being focused on them, with the new NHS Outcomes Framework including an indicator on reducing unplanned hospital admissions in under-19s for asthma, diabetes and epilepsy.

Despite the publication of extensive guidance, many of the articles included here show current provision to be generally falling some way short of best practice models. Similar concerns are evident in relation to transition planning, which now takes on even greater significance as enhanced treatment strategies have led to substantial improvements in life expectancy for young people with life-limiting conditions. Improving services for young people with long-term conditions must therefore remain a key priority for reformed health services. This is not just essential for their immediate quality of life. Establishing good health management in adolescence can help those affected to manage their condition far more effectively over their whole life course. This should also help to reduce demands and service costs in the longer term.

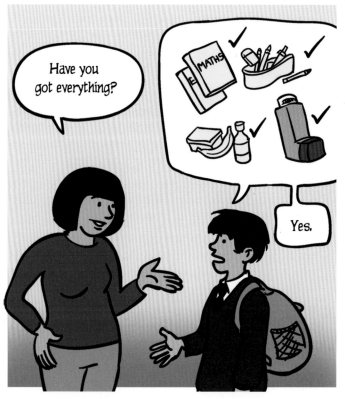

Latest data on long-term conditions

Statistics on the prevalence of selected long-term health conditions.

Asthma[2]

⇨ Around 1.1 million children and young people (one in 11) in the UK have asthma, making it the most common long-term medical condition.

⇨ On average, there are two children with asthma in every classroom, with the UK having one of the highest prevalence rates of asthma symptoms for children worldwide.

⇨ One in eight children with asthma symptoms experience attacks so severe that they can't speak.

⇨ The number of hospital admissions in England among 10-19-year-olds because of asthma has increased by 27% since 2002/3 to just under 8,600 in 2009/10.

⇨ An estimated 75% of hospital admissions are preventable – and people without an asthma action plan are four times more likely to have an attack requiring emergency hospital treatment.

Cancer[3]

⇨ Around one in 500 children in the UK develop some form of cancer by the age of 14, making it the most common cause of death from disease for children and young people.

⇨ Nearly 950 adolescents aged ten to 19 were diagnosed with cancer in England in 2008.

⇨ Rates for newly diagnosed cases (per 100,000 population) are higher among males and increase with age across the whole life course – in 2008, from a rate of 13.2 among boys aged 10-14 to 30.5 for young men aged 20-24.

1   Health Behaviour in School-aged Children (HBSC) – England National Report, University of Hertfordshire, 2011.

2   Most of the data here are taken from Key facts and statistics, Asthma UK (online) accessed 16 February 2012. The data on hospital admissions are from Hospital Episode Statistics, NHS Information Centre, 2011.

3   Most of the data here are from Key Facts – Childhood Cancer, Cancer Research UK (online) accessed 16 February 2012. The data on survival rates are from Survival of Children, Teenagers and Young Adults with Cancer in England, National Cancer Intelligence Network, 2011.

⇨ Improved treatment strategies have led to substantial increases in survival rates for childhood cancers over the past 40 years – nearly eight out of ten children diagnosed with cancer now survive for at least five years, compared with fewer than three in ten in the late 1960s. However, five-year survival rates for leukaemias are 25% higher for children aged 0-14 at diagnosis than for older adolescents and young adults aged 15-24.

Diabetes[4]

⇨ Around 29,000 children and young people in the UK have diabetes, with about 26,500 of them having Type 1 diabetes, 500 having Type 2 diabetes, and a further 2,000 with diabetes whose diagnosis is unknown.

⇨ The current estimate of prevalence of Type 1 diabetes in the UK is one per 700-1,000 children and young people, with the peak age for diagnosis being between ten and 14 years of age.

⇨ The number of hospital admissions in England among ten- to 19-year-olds because of diabetes has increased by 31% since 2002/3 to just under 7,600 in 2009/10.

⇨ Type 2 diabetes is now being diagnosed more frequently in younger overweight people and is most prevalent among children and young people of South Asian origin.

⇨ Obesity accounts for 80-85% of the overall risk of developing Type 2 diabetes and underlies the number of people diagnosed in the UK doubling from 1.4 million in 1996 to 2.9 million today. Latest forecasts suggest that over four million people will have diabetes by 2025.

Epilepsy[5]

⇨ Some 600,000 people in the UK have epilepsy – around 1% of the population – with young people under 18 accounting for around 10% of this total.

⇨ There were just over 5,400 hospital admissions among 10-19-year-olds in England for epilepsy in 2009/10 – an increase of 19% since 2002/3.

⇨ Many adolescents with epilepsy will 'grow out of it' in adult life.

February 2012

⇨ The above information is reprinted with kind permission from the Association for Young People's Health. Please visit www.ayph.org.uk for further information.

© *2012 Association for Young People's Health*

---

4   Most of the data here are taken from Diabetes in the UK 2011/2012: Key statistics on diabetes, Diabetes UK, 2011. The data on hospital admissions are from Hospital Episode Statistics, NHS Information Centre, 2011.

5   The first data here are from Epilepsy facts, figures and terminology, Epilepsy Action (online) and For teenagers, Young Epilepsy (online) – both accessed 16 February 2012. The data on hospital admissions are from Hospital Episode Statistics, NHS Information Centre, 2011.

Age	Type 1		Type 2		Other types		Total	
	Number	Per cent	Number	Per cent	Number	Per cent	Number	Per cent
0-4	827	4.0	0	0.0	31	9.7	858	4.1
5-9	3,920	19.1	6	1.8	34	10.6	3,960	18.7
10-14	8,715	42.5	128	39.1	114	35.6	8,957	42.2
15-17	7,026	34.3	194	59.1	141	44.1	7,361	34.8
Total	20,488	100	328	100	320	100	21,136	100

Source: Long-term conditions: AYPH Research Summary, *February 2012. AYPH*

Should we be worried about teenagers?

WHO/Europe has published the latest report from the Health Behaviour in School-aged Children (HBSC) study, based on interviews with over 200,000 young people. The study collects data and produces an international report every four years on the health, well-being, social environments and health behaviours of 11-, 13- and 15-year-old boys and girls.

Professor Candace Currie, the study's International Coordinator, explains some of its key findings, current trends and how HBSC began.

What are the major trends in the study's findings?

Gender differences

The continuing focus on issues relating to girls' body image and dieting from report to report is a concern. A lot of these gender differences appear to be really embedded and persistent, as are the inequalities related to affluence.

Girls tend to rate themselves poorly. They report that they think they're too fat; they don't feel very well; they have lower life satisfaction. We also know that, later on, some serious mental health problems emerge for young men, and we don't know if it's that girls just express themselves more in their teenage years. Perhaps boys feel unable to explain how they're feeling, or the prevailing culture is that you don't complain about how you feel if you're a boy. There's quite a lot of debate about what these gender differences really show.

Socialising online

There are some areas that have really changed in young peoples' lives. The whole emergence of electronic media and communications has changed. Going out in the evening is dropping and spending time on electronic communications is increasing. I think the whole way in which young people socialise is changing.

We have yet to see the impact of this change in social terms and I don't think it's necessarily going to be that easy to understand. While there's good evidence that children are at risk from cyber-bullying and so on, these forms of communication also give children who would normally find it difficult to make friends a new route. In this way they can identify people like them, befriend them and, in a gradual, uninhibited way, they can build groups. However, we really don't know the impact on being physically active. If your social life is sitting in your bedroom online, then you're not running around.

Risky behaviour

There also seem to be some quite strong trends in risk behaviour that are starting to emerge. We see big differences between the west and the east. In some aspects of risk taking, there's quite clear gender equalisation going on in the western countries, whereas there are still quite big gender gaps in drinking and sexual behaviour in the east. That's an oversimplification but it's giving us an insight. We're still in the process of trying to understand what these gender patterns signify.

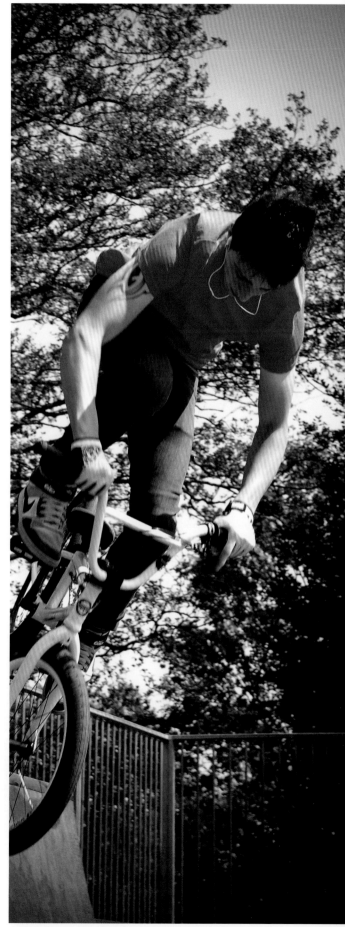

If girls are now behaving like boys in terms of risk, but they're still showing worse mental health outcomes, then that leads to the conclusion that girls are under a greater burden of potential ill health than boys. They're suffering at two levels. Previously, on the whole girls had healthier lifestyles but more mental health issues than boys. Now they're adopting risk behaviour that was previously in the male domain.

Should we be worried about teenagers?

Being worried is the wrong way of putting it! We should be paying attention to them and listening to them. It's well known that parental support is crucial for happy children and the development of well-being, but often, as children emerge into their teenage years and the relationship becomes more challenging in some cases, there's a tendency for parents to stand back and say, oh, well, they're spending more time with their friends and our role might not be so great.

Need for support within the family

But actually you'll see there's a big variation between countries in how much time they spend out with friends and how easy they find it to communicate with their parents, particularly with fathers. There's not a huge amount of cross-national variation with mothers, but there is with fathers. It's definitely evident that young people who have good parental support do better. What we need to pay attention to, is the fact that young people need to talk; they need guidance and support and they still need to be embraced within the family. It's less about being worried about them from a distance and more about thinking how we can support them through these years when their lives are changing.

How can we support adolescents?

Some things are quite concerning: the mental health changes that happen and particularly how that's affected by affluence, and also

we see these emerging gender differences. So we have to ask ourselves what it is about society that's giving less support to young people who are less affluent, or less support to girls for that matter. We have to ask ourselves what we need to do to provide a supportive environment so young people can grow up and have positive health. It's not just so that they're healthy adults, but so that they're happy healthy adolescents, including being happy at school and getting good grades, making friends and becoming socially skilled. They need support for that.

2 May 2012

⇨ The above information is reprinted with kind permission from the World Health Organization (WHO). Please visit www.euro.who.int for further information.

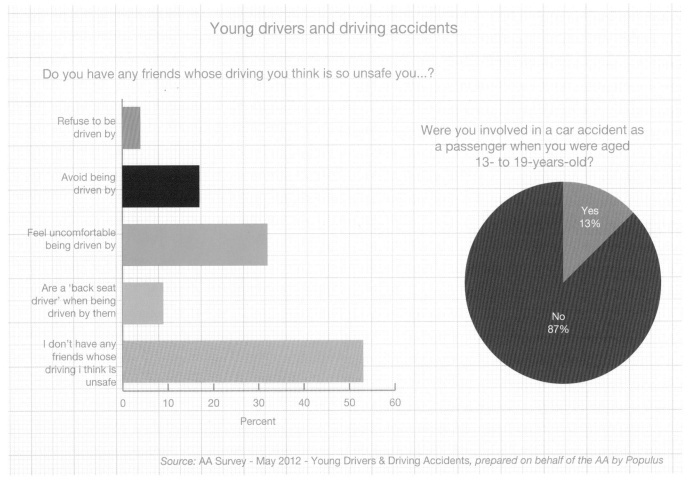

Young drivers and driving accidents

Do you have any friends whose driving you think is so unsafe you...?

Were you involved in a car accident as a passenger when you were aged 13- to 19-years-old?

Yes 13%

No 87%

- Refuse to be driven by
- Avoid being driven by
- Feel uncomfortable being driven by
- Are a 'back seat driver' when being driven by them
- I don't have any friends whose driving i think is unsafe

0 10 20 30 40 50 60

Percent

Source: AA Survey - May 2012 - Young Drivers & Driving Accidents, *prepared on behalf of the AA by Populus*

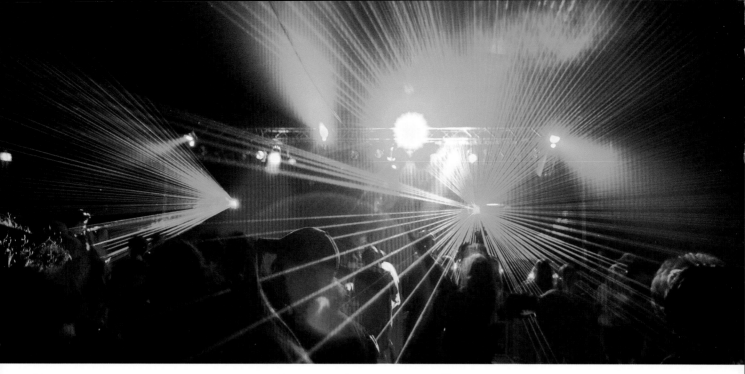

Does your mother know?

Staying out late and risky behaviours among ten- to 15-year-olds.

By Maria Iacovou

Throughout the ages, parents have fretted about how much control they should be exercising over the whereabouts of their teenage children. This issue has become particularly relevant in contemporary Britain, against the backdrop of the riots of 2011, with 'poor parenting' being blamed in some quarters for the disturbances, and with pronouncements by Parliament and regional police forces that parents should make sure they 'know where their children are' at night.

This article uses data from the youth questionnaire of Understanding Society, which asks children aged ten to 15 how frequently they have stayed out past 9pm without their parents knowing their whereabouts, over the past month. We also explore whether this is a 'bad thing', and examine whether there are differences between boys and girls, or between different age groups. In what follows, we sometimes abbreviate 'staying out past 9pm without your parents knowing where you are' as 'staying out late' but all the analysis relates to the same question.

A substantial minority report having done this even once in the past month (21% of boys and 15% of girls), with a much smaller proportion (4% of boys and 2% of girls) who report having done it frequently (ten or more times in the past month). As one would expect, it is much more common for older children to stay out after 9pm without their parents knowing where they are; it is also more common among boys. But even among 15-year-olds, only a minority (36% of boys and 24% of girls) say they have been out after 9pm without their parents knowing where they are.

The question is whether staying out late without parents knowing is a 'problem behaviour' or simply a manifestation of the fact that children become more independent, and

their parents trust them more to make their own decisions, as they reach their mid-teens.

We can say that staying out late is associated with other behaviours and characteristics which our society is inclined to define as problematic in young people. The table on page 12 demonstrates this for 15-year-olds: staying out late without your parents knowing is associated with visiting pubs or bars more often; with frequency of alcohol consumption; with smoking, and with cannabis use. These associations are visible for both boys and girls, though they are more pronounced for girls in relation to smoking and drinking.

Staying out late without your parents knowing is also related to emotional problems: boys are more at risk of conduct problems, whereas the relationship between staying out at night and both hyperactivity and poor self-esteem is much more pronounced for girls.

Clearly, these findings do not mean that staying out late without telling your parents where you are necessarily 'causes' a young person to start smoking or using recreational drugs, any more than smoking would 'cause' a young person to stay out at night. In order to examine why some groups of young people are more likely than others to stay out at night, it is more informative to look at other factors, such as where they live, what sorts of families they grew up in, and the quality of relationships within the family.

Analyses which examine or control for all these factors together reveal that (as we saw from earlier results) young men are more likely than young women to stay out late without telling their parents where they are; and the likelihood of doing this increases over the age range. Living in social housing or with a single mother also increases the probability, but living in a step family does not, and the number of siblings, grandparents or other people present in the household does not seem to have an effect. There are differences by nationality, with Scottish teenagers more likely than those living in England, Wales or Northern Ireland, to stay out late, and by ethnicity, with youngsters from Asian backgrounds less likely to stay out late than their white and African or Caribbean counterparts. There are also differences by the size of the community in which young people live: those living in hamlets and villages are less likely than those in towns and cities to go out at night without their parents knowing where they are. Young people who travel to school by independent means (on foot, bicycle, bus or train) are more likely than those who are taken to school by car to stay out at night. And finally, while family income has little effect on this particular aspect of youngsters' behaviour, family relationships are important: those who hardly ever talk about important matters with their mothers are more likely, and those who hardly ever quarrel with their mothers are less likely, to stay out late.

This analysis has shown that staying out late without telling your parents is associated with a number of risky or problem behaviours, and that the factors associated with staying out late are complex: some (such as geographical location) may relate to local entertainment opportunities; some (such as the mode of travel to school) probably relate to independence on the part of young people and trust on the part of parents; while others (most notably family relationships) demonstrate that social and emotional deprivation also play a role. Interestingly, while these sets of factors are all significantly related to staying out late, they are not all related to the problem behaviours discussed in the table opposite. While poor family relationships are related to both staying out late and to problem behaviours, other factors such as independent travel to school are related to staying out late, but not to problem behaviours.

This analysis is very much a first look at the issue of staying out late, and as such, leaves many questions unanswered. In particular, we have not addressed the distinction between staying out late without your parents knowing where you are, and staying out late at all. In addition, for young people who stay out late without their parents knowing where they are, there may be a distinction between those who

do this with and without their parents' consent. At present, these questions cannot be answered using data from Understanding Society, but as the sample matures, there may be scope for refining questions in this way.

Key findings

⇨ Staying out late without parents' knowledge was reported by 21% of boys and 15% of girls aged ten to 15. It was more common in boys and older children.

⇨ For 15-year-olds, staying out late is associated with risky behaviours: going to pubs, drinking alcohol and even using cannabis.

⇨ For 15-year-olds, staying out late is associated with conduct problems for boys and, for girls, poor self-esteem and hyperactivity.

⇨ The above information is reprinted with kind permission from the Institute for Social & Economic Research. Please visit www.understandingsociety.ac.uk for further information.

© 2013 Institute for Social & Economic Research (ISER)

Stayed out past 9pm without their parents' knowledge...		Never in past month	One or more times in past month	Three or more times in past month
		%	%	%
Go to a pub or bar once per week or more	Boys	5	7	14*
	Girls	4	6	11
Had alcohol more than once in past month	Boys	24	44 ***	56 ***
	Girls	25	51 ***	64 ***
Smoke	Boys	10	30 ***	33 ***
	Girls	18	41 ***	51 ***
Ever used cannabis	Boys	7	19 ***	38 ***
	Girls	5	15 **	37 ***
Score of six or more on conduct problems scale	Boys	6	10	19 ***
	Girls	2	6 **	7 *
Score of seven of more on hyperactivity scale	Boys	13	15	15
	Girls	12	24 ***	26 **
Poor self-esteem	Boys	18	21	23
	Girls	25	37*	32

Notes: Based on a sample of 651 boys and 662 girls aged 15, from Waves one and two of the Understanding Society youth sample. Asterisks denote figures where those staying out one or more, or three or more, times in the past month are statistically different from those not staying out. * significant at 10% level; ** significant at 5% level; *** significant at 1% level.

Children and young people with anxiety

This information resource has been produced by Catherine O'Neill for Anxiety UK. Anxiety UK would like to thank all of the parents who contributed and the professional expertise and guidance of Dr Sam Cartwright-Hatton and Dr Gillian Harris.

Introduction

It can often be difficult to discuss how you feel with other people, especially if you think that no one else feels the same, or that they won't understand. You may feel that you don't fully understand what is happening to you, which can make it very hard to explain to others exactly what you are going through. Often, experiencing anxiety can leave you feeling tired, upset and frustrated. This can make you feel that you are unable to cope or that there is nothing that you can do to improve your situation.

Anxiety can affect us all in very different ways. Experiences of anxiety can vary greatly from person to person and no two people are the same. If you feel that any of the experiences or symptoms described on these pages apply to you, then we may be able to help.

Something you should remember – anxiety is extremely common; we all experience it at times (perhaps when we have a deadline at work, or a test), in fact a recent study has suggested that 15% of young people have an episode of anxiety at some point. That means in the average class there will be five people who have experienced anxiety!

What is anxiety?

First of all, anxiety is completely normal! It is something that we all experience to some degree. Anxiety is useful to us as it tells us that something is dangerous and that we need to be careful. However, if

anxiety gets out of control or stops you from doing everyday things, then this can lead to us feeling unhappy, upset and frustrated.

Here are some examples of how you might feel if you are anxious:

⇨ Worried.

⇨ Upset.

⇨ Feeling sick.

⇨ Feeling shaky/dizzy.

⇨ Feeling like you might faint/pass out.

⇨ Thinking unpleasant thoughts.

⇨ Thinking that you might 'go crazy'.

When anxiety gets really strong, you might experience what we call a 'panic attack'.

This is when your body is getting ready to fight, freeze or to run away from the situation that we are viewing as dangerous. This is known as the fight, flight or freeze response.

Again, it can be quite scary to experience, although we know that it will not hurt you.

One of the ways to reduce the anxiety that you are feeling is to understand it

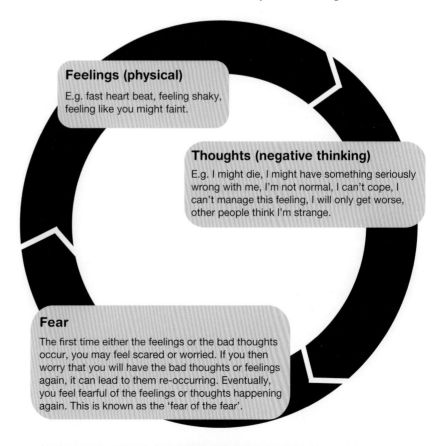

Feelings (physical)
E.g. fast heart beat, feeling shaky, feeling like you might faint.

Thoughts (negative thinking)
E.g. I might die, I might have something seriously wrong with me, I'm not normal, I can't cope, I can't manage this feeling, I will only get worse, other people think I'm strange.

Fear
The first time either the feelings or the bad thoughts occur, you may feel scared or worried. If you then worry that you will have the bad thoughts or feelings again, it can lead to them re-occurring. Eventually, you feel fearful of the feelings or thoughts happening again. This is known as the 'fear of the fear'.

better. By understanding how anxiety works, you can then understand why you feel that way (so that it is not so scary!) The diagram on page 13 can help to explain what happens when we get anxious. What it is saying is that with anxiety you can get into a vicious circle; your thoughts go round and round in your head – these impact on how you act and the things you do (for example, if you are feeling socially anxious you may avoid being around groups of people because you think they may judge you).

The 'fear of the fear' often makes us feel worse as we are literally on edge waiting for bad feelings to happen; we stop doing things that we link with the negative (bad) feelings or thoughts. This is called avoidance. The more that we avoid the thing that we link with feeling bad, the more we think of it as being dangerous.

This means that the next time we have to face the situation or event, our body tells us that it is dangerous and the fight, flight or freeze response kicks in. We feel that we either need to run away from the 'dangerous' thing, fight it or we feel that our body is frozen to the spot.

'The 'fear of the fear' often makes us feel worse as we are literally on edge waiting for bad feelings to happen'

Either way, our body is not happy when we feel all of these horrible feelings and think horrible things. By understanding why we feel this way, we can then take away the 'scared' feeling because we know that it is just our body reacting to something that it thinks is scary, even though it is actually harmless. No one ever died from having anxiety!

Case study – one girl's experience of anxiety

I have had agoraphobia since I was eight years old. No one noticed there was anything wrong until it got so bad that I couldn't go to school. I have been unable to attend school for about seven months and I have only just started getting the help I need. I want to go back to school to see

my friends but I worry that everyone will ask me loads of questions. My friend has been telling people at school that I'm dead. She has also been making up lies about me and telling my two best friends that I hate them and that I keep saying things about them behind their backs. My mum said she is not going to send me back to school until next year (the end of year 11) so that I can do my exams; however, because I have missed a year, I now have to stay on to sixth form. I am worrying about so many things at the moment and I have so much homework to do. I am also very worried about what people are saying about me at school. My agoraphobia has got so bad that I'm not even going outside now; most of the time I can't even leave my room. I want to be able to go out to places and to go back to school. I want to see my friends again and I would like to do the dance class that I started; however, at the moment I can't even leave the house without feeling that I will faint. My dad keeps saying there is nothing wrong with me and that I should be in school. My agoraphobia got really bad over Christmas as we had to go to my nan's on Boxing Day. I nearly fainted when I walked into the house. Not many people believe that I have agoraphobia and not a lot of people understand what agoraphobia is so I don't really have anyone to talk to.

Getting help and support

The good news is that anxiety is treatable! This means that there are things that can be done to reduce feelings of anxiety. The first step is to speak to someone that you trust about how you are feeling. This could be a teacher, a parent, a relative or another adult or friend that you trust. Talking to someone will reduce the pressure of anxiety and stress, it may also help you to realise that you are not alone in how you are feeling.

Talking to others

Often, because the anxious feelings and thoughts are so bad, we don't want to tell anyone how we feel as we believe that they might not understand or they might laugh at us.

However, this is the best way to get help to change how you feel. Talking to someone about how you feel can help.

⇨ Choose someone that you trust; for example, a parent/family member/teacher, etc.

⇨ Tell them how you have been feeling and try to give them an example so that they understand clearly how your problem is affecting you.

⇨ If you are finding it hard to talk about your anxiety, try writing your problem down or showing someone this article.

⇨ Remember: it is OK to be upset and it is OK to ask for help.

Once you have spoken to someone, they will be able to get help for you. You can also call Anxiety UK Helpline number: 08444 775 774 to talk to someone in complete confidence. We have included a list of telephone numbers of organisations that work with young people at the end of this article.

Email support/instant messaging

Many people want support to help them decide what information they need to manage their anxiety. If you are affected by an anxiety condition and want to email for information or to allow us to point you in the best direction to get some help, please email us at support@phobics-society.org.uk. The service is free and we will not tell anyone about the information that you put into the email. This service is not a counselling service but we can point you in the direction of further help and support. Don't be worried about anything that you write in the email – all of the volunteers who answer the emails are trained to deal with anxiety and also have personal experience of anxiety so they understand what you are feeling. We also have a new instant messaging service where you can get access to information instantly; this is also free and can be accessed via the 'live help' button on our website (http://www.phobicssociety.org.uk/youngpeople.php).

Professionals

Sometimes, although we are trying to reduce our anxiety by undertaking certain activities on our own initiative, this might not be enough to help us cope with the anxiety and we may need to gain the help of a professional. A professional is someone who can discuss how you are feeling and can help you to put things into place to make your problems manageable. All of the professionals you may encounter have to make sure that they keep all of the information that you tell them private so don't worry about anyone finding out that you have anxiety.

'There are things that can be done to reduce feelings of anxiety. The first step is to speak to someone that you trust about how you are feeling'

The following professionals are ones which you may come into contact with when trying to access help:

Your doctor/GP

Don't worry about talking to your doctor about anxiety, it is one of the most common problems that people go to see them about! Your GP can also help you access different sources of support as they have lots of contacts in your area.

School nurse

Most schools have a school nurse who should know about anxiety. They can be a good person to talk to as they are quite often independent from the school and your family and can help you to get any help and support you ask for.

Counsellors

A counsellor is someone who you are able to talk to about how you are feeling with your anxiety. They will provide you with a safe place to talk about your experiences. Most counsellors will help you to look at where these feelings have come from and why you may be feeling the way that you do. Going to see a counsellor does not mean that you are 'mad' or that you will 'go crazy'! Lots of people see counsellors to help them with all sorts of problems. Friends finding out that you are seeing a counsellor is often a very big worry for many young people. What will they say? Will they think that I am weird? Will they tease me? Will they understand?

The best thing about seeing a counsellor is that it is completely confidential. This means that the counsellor is not allowed to talk about what you say to them to anyone. Therefore, the only person who can tell the people at school that you are seeing a counsellor is you.

Cognitive behaviour therapists (CBT)

This sounds like a very complicated therapy but actually it is very simple! 'Cognitive' just means our thoughts and the things that we are thinking, whereas 'Behaviour' means exactly what it says on the tin, that is the acts that we carry out and the things that we do. This type of therapist will look at how you are feeling in the 'here and now' and how the problem can be managed more effectively. They will look at getting you to practise certain behaviours and thoughts to try to improve what you are feeling. Often the things that you are asked to practise are the opposite to what the anxiety wants you to do. This makes it a bit harder but it is like riding a bike – the more that you practise, the less you fall off!

Hypnotherapists

Hypnotherapy is not about getting you up on a stage where you will be made to do all sorts of silly things in front of an audience! It is completely different to stage hypnotism and clinical hypnotherapists will aim to make you feel relaxed and safe whilst they use visualisation techniques (e.g. asking you to picture events going well and places that you feel safe) to improve your anxiety.

Remember: anxiety is treatable and it doesn't have to keep making you feel unhappy. Things can change and you can control your stress and anxiety.

Other places where you can get help and support

ChildLine

ChildLine is the UK's free, 24-hour helpline for children in distress. Trained volunteer counsellors comfort, advise and protect children and young people who may feel they have nowhere else to turn.

Website: www.childline.org.uk

Helpline: 0800 1111 (Freephone)

NSPCC

NSPCC works to support children and young people across the UK. They have a helpline (in conjunction with ChildLine) and a range of websites that offer interactive advice and support.

Websites: www.nspcc.org.uk

www.there4me.com

Helpline: 0800 1111 (Freephone)

CALM (Campaign Against Living Miserably)

CALM works with young men and provides information advice and support via a free helpline and website. They also offer free downloads and chat rooms for those that need support.

Website: www.thecalmzone.net

Helpline: 0800 585858

Youngminds

Youngminds focus on the mental health issues of children, recognising that many children have troublesome worries and fears.

Website: www.youngminds.org.uk/young-people

Kooth

Kooth is a free, anonymous, safe, secure and confidential online counselling and advice service. It is available to 15-25-year-olds who live in Stockport, St Helens, Wirral, Halton, Warrington, Wigan, Knowsley and Warwickshire.

Website: www.kooth.com

⇨ The above information is reprinted with kind permission from Anxiety UK. Please visit www.anxietyuk.org.uk for further information.

© Anxiety UK 2013

Exam stress

Sometimes exams can leave you feeling overwhelmed and unable to cope. The good news is the stress can be managed and help is available.

If you're stressed about exams you can talk to ChildLine

The pressure to revise and do well in exams, whether it's from your parents or your teachers can be very stressful.

You might be worried you are going to fail or that you won't get the grades you need for the job or course you want.

If you are stressed about anything to do with exams, you can always talk to ChildLine – they are there for you no matter how big or small your worry.

You can speak to a counsellor by calling free on 0800 1111 or through 1-2-1 chat online, or email. Or get support from other young people on the message boards.

The pressure of exams can make you anxious

Anxiety can sometimes make you feel tired, upset, worried, shaky, light-headed, frustrated or feeling like you might 'go crazy'. It can also present itself as a panic attack, or make you feel like you might be sick.

Anxiety or stress can be a result of something specific (like writing exams) or you could be feeling stressed for no specific reason, which is normal and OK too.

Coping with stress

It can seem scary at first to talk about stress or anxiety, as you might feel like nobody else is feeling this way or would understand. This often makes the stress worse.

If you think you might be experiencing anxiety or stress, talking about it with someone you trust can be the next step. Talking about how you are feeling can reduce the pressure and help you to feel more in control.

Problems at home or school can make it hard to concentrate

If your family are arguing or going through a tough time themselves, it can make finding time to revise and concentrate even more difficult. Things affecting your concentration could include:

⇨ Family arguing

⇨ Problems with your girlfriend/ boyfriend

⇨ Feeling like you want to hurt yourself

⇨ Bullying

⇨ Depression and feeling sad

⇨ Having to look after people in your family.

If you feel any of these problems are affecting your work, it is important to tell someone how you feel. This could be a teacher or a trusted friend. In some serious circumstances, your school might

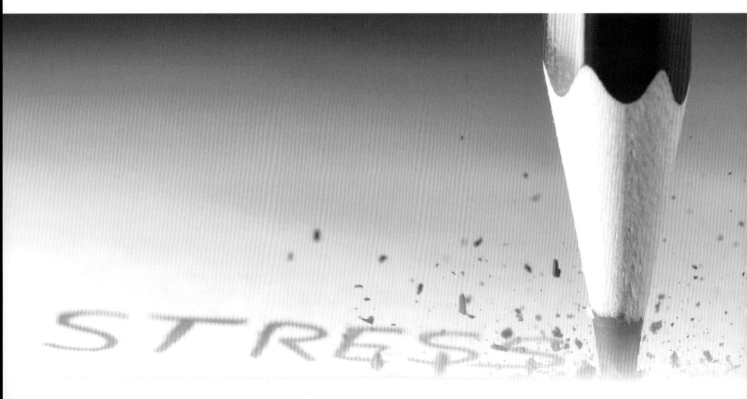

be able to make exceptions which they can discuss with you.

What is exam stress?

Exam stress starts when you feel you can't cope with revision, sitting exams or pressure from your school or family. If you feel stressed about taking exams you aren't alone in feeling like this – lots of other young people experience anxiety at exam time.

If you feel overwhelmed by exam stress you can talk to ChildLine to get help and support to find a way to cope with the anxiety and worry.

I'm scared I'm going to fail my exams

'I have my GCSEs coming up, and I am getting so stressed and worried that I'm going to do awful in them.'

'I can't cope with A-levels any more, I get so worked up that I just cry.'

When we feel anxious, we often give ourselves negative messages such as, 'I can't do this', 'I'm useless' and 'I'm going to fail'. It can be difficult but try and replace these with encouraging thoughts such as: 'this is just anxiety, it can't harm me' and, 'relax, concentrate; it is going to be OK'. By picturing how you would like things to go, this can help you feel more positive. For example, try to imagine yourself turning up to an exam feeling confident and relaxed. You turn over your paper, write down what you do know and come away knowing you tried your best on the day.

If I don't get the grades I need, it'll ruin everything

'I'm about to start my very important GCSEs. I'm worried that I won't revise for them and ruin my future

'My head's all over the place, I don't know what I'm gonna do if I don't get in.'

It can sometimes feel like the whole of your future depends on what grades you get. First of all, try not to panic. You have a while until exam results come out. Even if you don't get the results you need or expect, you still have options and can get help with any decisions you have to make.

Remember, exams are important – but they are not the only key to a successful future.

Everyone expects me to do really well, it's stressing me out

'I am really nervous. Everyone expects me to do really well but being put under pressure I feel like I am going to fail.'

There can be a lot of pressure on young people to do well in exams which can cause a lot of stress and anxiety. You might have been predicted certain grades or put into a higher set, and feel if you don't get the grade you'll let your teachers or parents down.

Talking to your parents or teachers about how you feel could really help. They might not be aware of how their attitude toward your exams is putting pressure on you. Take a look at the message boards and get advice from other young people who may be in the same situation.

My friends never revise, yet they always do better than me

'You're judged if u do awful, you're put into sets and I did awful last year, I need to up my game.'

'Everyone is better than me, I feel so stupid.'

During exam time, it's easy to start comparing your own revision

or performance with that of your friends. Some people in your class might be bragging about how easy they are finding it all whilst you might be struggling.

Not understanding something at first does not mean you are thick or stupid. Everyone learns in different ways and you have to find a way that suits you. Try and focus on your own work and not put yourself down.

Some people are more academic than others, but this doesn't mean your future won't be successful. Nobody is good at everything. Where some people might fail, you could be the one to shine through and succeed.

I'm worried about sitting the exam

There is nothing wrong with being worried about the actual exam, it's very normal. The more prepared we are, the more confident we feel in being able to cope.

There are lots of things you can do to get ready for your exams, whether you are taking GCSEs, A-Levels, Scottish Highers or another kind of exam, it's important to find what works for you.

Your teacher is also there to support you. Don't be ashamed to ask for help and talk to them about how you feel. Together you might be able to find a solution which will help you feel better.

⇨ The above article is reprinted with kind permission from ChildLine. Whatever your worry, you can call ChildLine free on 0800 1111 or chat to a counsellor online. Visit www. childline.org.uk for information and support.

© ChildLine 2013

Depression in children and young people

Published by Bupa's Health Information Team.

Depression is a condition in which people may have low mood, a loss of interest in everyday activities, feelings of low self-worth, a lack of energy and poor concentration, all of which last a long time. Depression in children and young people can often come back (recur) and continue into adulthood. It's therefore important to treat the condition as early as possible.

About depression in children and young people

Around one in 100 children are affected by depression before they reach puberty and three in every 100 teenagers are affected. Depression is twice as common in girls than in boys.

All children feel sad or miserable from time to time, but these feelings often pass. Depression can make your child feel sad or low for a long period of time and it can interfere with his or her life.

There are three levels of depression that are classified according to the symptoms your child has.

⇨ Mild depression can cause your child to feel unhappy, but won't stop him or her from leading a normal life. Your child may find everyday things difficult to do and less worthwhile. Simple lifestyle changes can help your child recover from mild depression.

⇨ Moderate depression can have a significant impact on your child's life. It can make him or her feel constantly miserable and low. Your child should visit a GP, as changes in lifestyle alone are unlikely to help.

⇨ Severe depression can cause your child to have constant negative thoughts and feel like he or she isn't able to cope. It's important that your child visits a doctor immediately, as he or she may have suicidal thoughts.

Around one in ten children who have depression recover within three months. After a year, half of all children with depression get better.

Symptoms of depression in children and young people

The symptoms of depression can vary from person to person. Some of the most common symptoms include:

⇨ constantly having a low mood and being irritable

⇨ losing interest in everyday activities

⇨ feeling guilty or bad, being self-critical and self-blaming

⇨ feeling hopeless or helpless

⇨ crying a lot

⇨ feeling unhappy for most of the day

⇨ lacking self-esteem and not wanting to see friends or family

⇨ problems sleeping

⇨ tiredness and lack of energy

⇨ difficulty concentrating

⇨ loss of confidence

⇨ changes in appetite

⇨ frequent aches and pains

⇨ having thoughts about death or suicide.

It can sometimes be difficult to tell if a young person has symptoms of depression or is showing signs of normal adolescent development. Generally, children are said to have depression if they have symptoms for two weeks or longer.

These symptoms may be caused by problems other than depression. If your child has any of these symptoms, see your GP for advice.

'Around one in 100 children are affected by depression before they reach puberty'

Complications of depression in children and young people

Severe depression is associated with self-harm and suicide, so it's important that you look out for changes in your child's mood.

Causes of depression in children and young people

Depression in children and young people is normally caused by a number of factors, including:

⇨ family problems or parents splitting up

⇨ death of a relative, friend or someone close

⇨ abuse

⇨ bullying

⇨ neglect

⇨ long-term health problems or serious illness

⇨ problems at school, such as low grades

⇨ a major life change such as moving house

⇨ friendship or boyfriend/girlfriend relationship problems

⇨ alcohol or drug use.

Depression is thought to run in families and a child with a close relative who has depression is more likely to get depression themselves. It's also linked to changes in how your child's brain works. Chemical changes are thought to happen in the part of your child's brain that controls mood and this causes the symptoms of depression.

If your child has had depression, his or her risk of having depression again within five years is higher than a child who hasn't had depression. However, most children and young people who have depression will go on to lead a normal adult life.

Diagnosis of depression in children and young people

It's important to seek medical help early if you think your child has depression. Your child's GP is a good first point of contact. He or she may suggest that your child goes to a child and adolescent mental health service for help. Your child may do a number of psychological and medical tests to see if any other medical condition is causing your child's symptoms.

Many young people who have depression get better by themselves, but if your child has severe depression your GP may refer him or her to see a psychiatrist, a doctor who specialises in mental health problems, or a clinical psychologist who can talk with your child about his or her problems.

Treatment of depression in children and young people

There are a number of treatments available for depression. Your doctor will be able to advise you which type of treatment is most suitable for your child.

Self-help

If your child has mild depression, there are a number of things he or she can do to help. For example, regular exercise, such as walking, running, swimming or cycling can help your child to feel better. Your child's doctor may advise him or her

to follow an exercise programme. It's also important that your child eats a healthy, well-balanced diet.

Providing support to your child is also very important. For example, you could try talking to your child about his or her problems and give some reassurance that you will help him or her to get better.

Talking therapies

Your child's doctor may advise that he or she has a talking therapy. However, the type of talking therapy your child has will depend on its availability, his or her preferences, and what is most suitable.

Counselling involves your child talking to a therapist about his or her problems. In these sessions, the counsellor won't offer advice or treatment, but will ask your child questions to help resolve his or her worries. Counsellors can sometimes help by working with you and your child's school.

Cognitive behavioural therapy (CBT) can help your child to change his or her behaviour and negative thoughts and feelings. Your child may be able to have cognitive behavioural therapy individually or in a group with other people the same age. Your child's doctor will be able to advise you about what is most suitable.

Interpersonal therapy involves your child talking with a therapist about any relationship problems he or she may have with friends, family or people at school. Your child's therapist may be able to help your child to solve or manage his or her problems.

Family therapy is a type of treatment that involves you and your child working together. You will meet with a therapist and your child will talk about any problems he or she is having. It's important that you and any other family members who are involved with your child go to the sessions together.

Medicines

Antidepressant medication will only be prescribed to your child if he or she has severe depression, or if his or her symptoms don't go away. Your child's doctor may advise that he or she takes an antidepressant called

fluoxetine (Prozac) as well as having a talking therapy.

Your child will be monitored weekly for the first four weeks of treatment and then regularly after. Your child's doctor will give you and your child information about any possible side-effects of the medicine and how long the treatment should last.

If your child doesn't feel better after taking fluoxetine, then he or she may be prescribed a different antidepressant such as sertraline or citalopram, but this is rare. Always ask your doctor for advice and read the patient information leaflet that comes with the medicine.

'It's important to seek medical help early if you think your child has depression'

Your child will need to take the antidepressant medication for six months after he or she feels better.

Hospital treatment

Most children and young people who have depression get better without needing hospital treatment. However, if your child has suicidal thoughts or his or her doctor is concerned about self-harm, he or she may need to go into hospital. If this happens, your child's doctor will be able to give you and your child more information and advice.

Complementary therapies

St John's wort is often used by adults as an alternative to antidepressants. However, children shouldn't use St John's wort for the treatment of depression as the safety of the herbal remedy is unknown in children.

April 2011

⇨ The above information is reprinted with kind permission from Bupa. Please visit www.bupa.co.uk for further information.

Depression linked to late-night screen use

Recent research from the United States shows that late-night exposure to light from a television or computer screen could be a risk factor for depression.

According to a team of neuroscientists at Ohio State University Medical Center, sitting in front of a screen just before bed, or leaving it on when you fall asleep could boost your chances of becoming depressed.

Late-night exposure to artificial light has already been identified as a risk factor for breast cancer and obesity, but little is yet known about its link with mood disorders like depression.

For the purposes of the study, which was partly funded by the US Department of Defense, the researchers exposed hamsters to dim light at night.

They then recorded behavioural changes and differences in brain chemistry that are linked to depression in humans.

The link could be a factor in surging depression rates during the past 50 years, which have coincided with a rise in people's exposure to artificial light late at night.

According to lead author Tracy Bedrosian, the links were particularly pronounced in women, who are twice as likely to become depressed as men.

She said that the team's results from the study in hamsters were consistent with what is already known about depression in humans.

Writing in the journal *Molecular Psychiatry*, Bedrosian's team described an experiment in which hamsters were exposed to dim light at night equivalent to a television screen in a darkened room for a period of four weeks.

A control group was exposed to a typical day-night light cycle.

The experimental group was observed to be less active and showed much less interest than usual in drinking sugar water, symptoms with mimic those of depression in humans.

The hamsters exposed to late-night light also showed marked changes in their hippocampus, a part of the brain affected in humans with depression.

They also produced more of a chemical messenger that is mobilised when the body is injured or infected – a protein known as tumour necrosis factor (TNF).

According to study co-author Randy Nelson, TNF causes inflammation in its attempts to repair damage to the body, which makes the relationship between dim light at night and increased TNF production particularly meaningful.

He said that previous studies have found a strong association in people between chronic inflammation and depression.

While blocking the TNF with a drug dampened its production, the other effects remained.

However, the symptoms were found to be reversible, because when the experimental group of hamsters was returned to a normal light-dark cycle, their brains returned to normal within about two weeks.

Bedrosian said that people who stay up late in front of the television and computer could potentially reverse the damage by minimising their exposure to artificial light at night.

24 July 2012

⇨ The above information is reprinted with kind permission from Healthcare Today. Please visit www.healthcare-today. co.uk for further information.

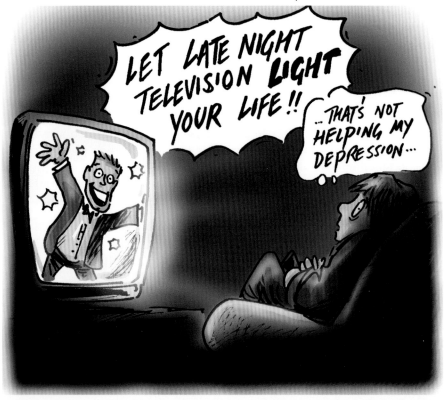

LET LATE NIGHT TELEVISION LIGHT YOUR LIFE !!

...THAT'S NOT HELPING MY DEPRESSION...

One in ten young people feel unable to cope with life

One in ten young people (ten per cent) feel they cannot cope with day-to-day life, warns a new report.

The Prince's Trust Youth Index reveals that young people not in employment, education or training (NEETs) are more than twice as likely to feel unable to cope as their peers.[1]

The report – based on interviews with 2,136 16 to 25-year-olds – also shows how more than one in five young people (22 per cent) did not have someone to talk to about their problems while they were growing up.

According to the research, NEET young people are significantly less likely to have had someone to talk to about their problems.[2]

Martina Milburn, chief executive of The Prince's Trust, said: 'A frightening number of unemployed young people feel unable to cope – and it is particularly tough for those who don't have a support network in place.

'We know at The Prince's Trust that it is often those from the most vulnerable backgrounds who end up furthest from the job market. Life can become a demoralising downward spiral – from a challenging childhood into life as a jobless adult. But, with the right support, we can help get these lives on track.'

The charity's fifth annual Youth Index – which gauges young people's well-being across a range of areas from family life to physical health – shows how NEETs are significantly less happy across all areas of their lives.

The report reveals that while 27 per cent of young people in work feel down or depressed 'always' or 'often', this increases to almost half (48 per cent) among NEETs.

Richard Parish, chief executive of the Royal Society for Public Health, said: 'The Youth Index clearly shows a worrying discrepancy between young people who are in work and those who are not. These unemployed young people need support to re-gain their self-worth and, ultimately, get them back in the workplace.

'With recent record-breaking youth unemployment – the work of charities like The Prince's Trust with vulnerable young people is more critical than ever.'

The Prince's Trust launched additional support for young people with mental health needs on its Team programme four years ago and has been increasing this support year-on-year ever since. More than 8,200 young people to date have benefited from the Working for Wellbeing project, which is funded by Zurich Community Trust.

The Prince's Trust provides a range of personal development programmes, pre-apprenticeship schemes and mentoring to help young people into jobs. Three in four young people supported by The Prince's Trust move into work, education or training.

For more information about how to help The Prince's Trust support more young people, visit www. princes-trust.org.uk/youthindex or follow The Trust on Facebook or Twitter www.facebook.com/ princes-trust / www.twitter.com/ princestrust.

2 January 2013

⇨ The above information is reprinted with kind permission from the Royal Society for Public Health. Please visit www.rsph.org.uk for further information.

© Royal Society for Public Health 2013

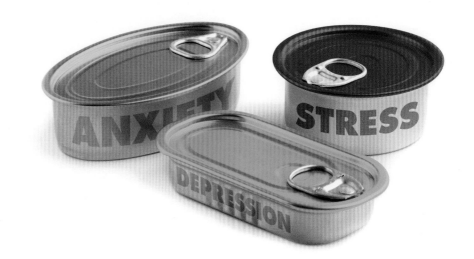

1 More than one in five (22 per cent) of NEET young people feel they cannot cope with day-to-day life.

2 31 per cent of NEET young people did not have someone to talk to about their problems while they were growing up.

The truth about self-harm

For young people and their friends and families.

Celia Richardson, Director of Communications at the Mental Health Foundation

Introduction

Self-harm is a very common problem, and many people are struggling to deal with it. Perhaps you feel or have felt the need to harm yourself. Perhaps you have been self-harming for some time. Or maybe you have a friend, brother or sister or a son or daughter who is self-harming, or someone you teach or work with is doing it and you need to know more.

This article is for anyone who wants to understand self-harm among young people – why it happens, how to deal with it, and how to recover from what can become a very destructive cycle.

Self-harm can be difficult to understand – both for those who do it and also for those who care about them. It is also a subject that has not received much attention up until now, and is still treated as 'taboo' by many. But it happens a lot more than people think. The most important thing to understand is that you can recover from the pattern of self-harm, and from feeling the urge to harm yourself.

Understanding self-harm

Many find it almost impossible to understand why young people harm themselves, and how it could possibly help them to feel better. By deliberately hurting their bodies, young people often say they can change their state of mind so that they can cope better with 'other' pain they are feeling. They may be using physical pain as a way of distracting themselves from emotional pain. Others are conscious of a sense of release. For some, especially those who feel emotionally scarred, it may be a way to 'wake up' in situations where they are so numb they can't feel anything. Overall, self-harm is a way of dealing with intense emotional pain.

Self-harm has a huge impact on the day-to-day life of those who do it. They will often try hard to keep what they're doing secret, and to hide their scars and bruises. But the burden of guilt and secrecy is difficult to carry. It can affect everything from what they wear to the kinds of sports and physical activities they take part in, as well as close physical relationships with others, including sexual relationships.

Ultimately, because young people who do it are all too aware of the stigma of self-harm, it can affect their relationships with friends and family and their sense of self-worth. Young people start self-

harming to cope with their problems and feelings, but it very soon creates other serious problems. It can set up an addictive pattern of behaviour, from which it can be very hard to break free.

What is self-harm?

The phrase 'self-harm' is used to describe a range of things that people do to themselves in a deliberate and usually hidden way. It can involve:

⇨ cutting

⇨ burning

⇨ scalding

⇨ banging or scratching one's own body

⇨ breaking bones

⇨ hair pulling

⇨ swallowing poisonous substances or objects.

Who does it?

Research shows that one in 15 young people in Britain have harmed themselves. Another way of looking at it is that there are probably two young people in every secondary school classroom who have done it at some time. This means it's a very common problem.

Most young people who harm themselves are aged between 11 and 25. The age at which most people start is 12, but some children as young as seven have been known to do it.

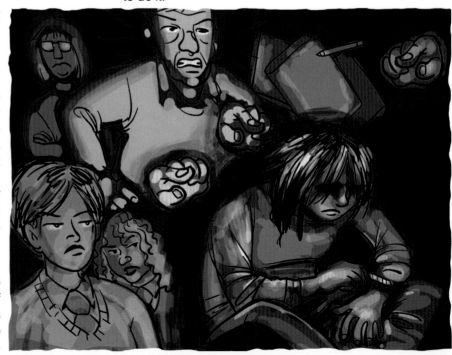

There is no such thing as a 'typical' young person who self-harms. About four times as many girls as boys do it. But it is also a serious problem among young men. Because they are more likely to do things like hitting themselves or breaking their own bones it can look as if they have had an accident, a fight or have been attacked.

Some very young children self-harm, and some adults too. Groups of people who are more vulnerable to self-harm than others include:

⇨ young people in residential settings like the armed forces, prison, sheltered housing or hostels and boarding schools

⇨ lesbian, gay, bisexual and transgender young people

⇨ young Asian women

⇨ young people with learning disabilities.

Why do young people self-harm?

As one young person put it, many people self-harm to 'get out the hurt, anger and pain' caused by pressures in their lives. They harm themselves because they don't know what else to do and because they don't have, or don't feel they have, any other options. For some young people, self-harm gives temporary relief and a sense of control over their lives. But it brings its own very serious problems.

When asked about the issues that led them to self-harm, young people most often said it was linked with:

⇨ Being bullied at school.

⇨ Not getting on with parents or other family members.

⇨ Stress and worry about school work and exams.

⇨ Feeling isolated.

⇨ Parents getting divorced.

⇨ Bereavement.

⇨ Unwanted pregnancy.

⇨ Experience of abuse earlier in childhood.

⇨ Current abuse – physical, sexual or verbal.

⇨ The self-harm or suicide of someone close to them.

⇨ Problems to do with sexuality.

⇨ Problems to do with race, culture or religion.

⇨ Low self-esteem.

⇨ Feelings of rejection socially or within their families.

Myths and stereotypes

There are lots of these attached to self-harm. This isn't surprising – myths and misunderstandings often arise when a problem is, like self-harm, poorly understood.

Negative stereotypes can be powerful. They need to be challenged because they stop young people from coming forward for help. They also mean that professionals, family and friends are much more likely to react in an inappropriate or hostile way to young people who self-harm.

Some of the most common stereotypes are that self-harm is about 'attention seeking'. Most self-harm is actually done in secret, for a long time and it can be very hard for young people to find enough courage to ask for help.

Self-harm is sometimes seen as a group activity – especially when young people are 'goths' or 'emos'. But it's very rarely a group activity. Young people told the Inquiry that they couldn't say how many people they knew who self-harmed, because no one wants to talk about it. The inquiry could find no evidence to support the belief that this behaviour may be part of a particular youth sub-culture.

⇨ The above information is reprinted with kind permission from the Mental Health Foundation. Please visit www. mentalhealth.org.uk for further information.

© *Mental Health Foundation 2013*

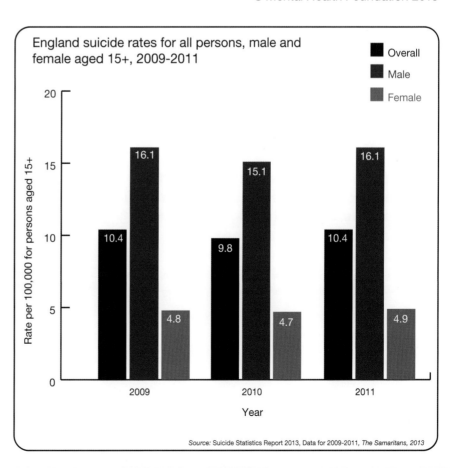

England suicide rates for all persons, male and female aged 15+, 2009-2011

Source: Suicide Statistics Report 2013, Data for 2009-2011, *The Samaritans, 2013*

Depression and fast food link confirmed

Eating fast foods such as hamburgers, hotdogs and pizza and baked commercial goods like fairy cakes, croissants and doughnuts is linked directly to depression, it has been confirmed.

The study, headed by scientists from the University of Las Palmas de Gran Canaria and the University of Granada, found that fast food consumers, compared to those who eat little or none, are 51% more likely to develop depression.

Published in the *Public Health Nutrition* journal, the results also found the more fast food consumed, the greater the risk of depression.

The study demonstrates that those participants who eat the most fast food and commercial baked goods are more likely to be single, less active and have poor dietary habits, which include eating less fruit, nuts, fish, vegetables and olive oil. Smoking and working more than 45 hours per week are other prevalent characteristics of this group.

'Depression affects 121 million people worldwide. This figure makes it one of the main global causes of disability-adjusted life year'

Of commercial baked goods, Almudena Sánchez-Villegas, lead author of the study, said: 'Even eating small quantities is linked to a significantly higher chance of developing depression.'

The study sample belonged to the SUN Project (University of Navarra Diet and Lifestyle Tracking Program). It consisted of 8,964 participants that had never been diagnosed with depression or taken antidepressants. They were assessed for an average of six months, and 493 were diagnosed with depression or started to take antidepressants.

'Participants who eat the most fast food and commercial baked goods are more likely to be single, less active and have poor dietary habits'

This new data supports the results of the SUN project in 2011, which were published in the *PLoS One* journal.

The project recorded 657 new cases of depression out of the 12,059 people analysed over more than six months. A 42% increase in the risk associated with fast food was found, which is lower than that found in the current study.

Sánchez-Villegas concludes that 'although more studies are necessary, the intake of this type of food should be controlled because of its implications on both health (obesity, cardiovascular diseases) and mental well-being'.

Depression affects 121 million people worldwide. This figure makes it one of the main global causes of disability-adjusted life year. Further still, in countries with low and medium income it is the leading cause.

However, little is known about the role that diet plays in developing depressive disorders. Previous studies suggest that certain nutrients have a preventative role. These include group B vitamins, omega-3 fatty acids and olive oil. Furthermore, a healthy diet such as that enjoyed in the Mediterranean has been linked to a lower risk of developing depression.

2 April 2012

⇨ The above information is reprinted with kind permission from *The Huffington Post*. Please visit www.huffingtonpost.com for further informtion.

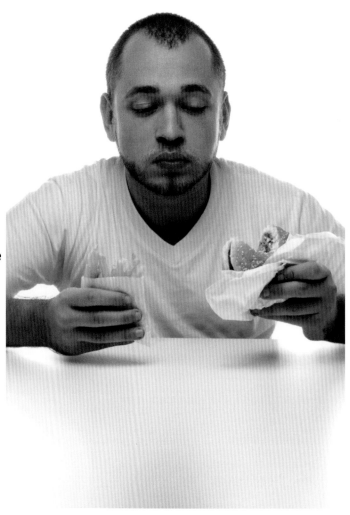

Improving mental health

Sometimes it can feel like we don't have any control over what we think or how we feel. But by making simple changes to our lives, we can make a real difference to our mental health. Feeling good is worth investing in – and the best thing is that these simple tips won't cost you much time or money.

Eat well, feel better

Did you know good food is good for your mood? It's not just your body you're feeding – your mind is affected by what you eat, too.

There is increasing evidence of a link between what we eat and how we feel. This is called the 'food – mood' connection. How we feel influences what we choose to eat or drink – and a healthy diet can protect our mental health.

How does food affect my mood?

Blood sugar

Glucose from the carbohydrate-containing foods we eat provides the brain's main source of fuel. Without this fuel, we can't think clearly.

Some carbs are better than others. Sugar, white pasta and biscuits will only give you a short burst of energy. You'll feel tired and grumpy when the sugar high wears off. 'Complex carbohydrates', such as wholegrains, beans and vegetables, are a better choice because they give you sustained energy.

If you eat lots of sugary foods, fizzy drinks and stimulants such as coffee, tea or alcohol, your blood sugar levels go up and down. This can make you irritable, anxious and dizzy, It can also lead to poor concentration and aggressive behaviour.

Protein

Proteins found mainly in meat, fish and soya products are broken down in the body to be used as amino acids, which are vital to good mental health. Brain messengers are made in the body from the proteins that we eat.

If we don't get enough amino acids, this can lead to feelings of depression, apathy, lack of motivation or tension.

Good fats

Essential fats, found mainly in oily fish, seeds and nuts, cannot be made within the body, so we have to get them from food. 60 per cent of the brain is made of fat, and the fats we eat directly affect its structure. A lack of omega-3 fatty acids has been linked to various mental health problems, including depression and lack of concentration.

Brain food: top tips

⇨ Don't skip meals. Eat three meals a day with two 'healthy' snacks (for example, fruit or yoghurt) in between.

⇨ Eat breakfast within an hour of waking up. Never skip breakfast.

⇨ Try to have at least five portions of fruit and vegetables every day.

⇨ Try to drink six to eight glasses of water every day.

Eat well on a budget

Good food doesn't have to break the bank. The Royal College of Psychiatrists has these tips for brain food on a budget.

1. Avoid ready meals and takeaways. They are usually bad for you and poor value for money.

2. Crisps, ice creams and sweets should be kept as an occasional treat.

3. Buy fruits and vegetables in season, when they're cheaper.

4. Buy fresh foods such as fruit, vegetables and meats in small amounts and more often since they go off easily.

5. Avoid tinned foods as they're usually more expensive. For example, dried beans and pasta are less expensive than canned beans and processed pasta.

6. Avoid fizzy drinks and fruit juices. They are often quite expensive. Use water and fruit instead.

7. Compare prices in local shops and supermarkets and take advantage of special offers.

8. Use 'generic' supermarket brands instead of classic brands. They often contain the same ingredients but are cheaper.

9. Cook and eat together with others and share the costs.

10. Make a shopping list and plan your food budget every week. If you feel you cannot do this on your own, ask for help.

Take time out

How many times have you been told to 'chill out', 'chillax' or 'stop stressing'? These are everyday phrases but taking time to relax is really important to maintain positive mental health.

Failing to take time to recharge your batteries and relax can contribute to some mental health problems such as anxiety or depression or make existing mental disorders worse. Relaxation therefore is key to maintaining positive mental well-being.

Whether you are at school, college or working, things can get on top of us all at certain times and relaxation is vital to help our minds and bodies switch off from those pressures.

Positive versus negative relaxation

There are ways to relax that are not so helpful in the long-term. Often it can be all too easy to turn to cigarettes, alcohol or even drugs as a 'quick fix' to wind down. But not only can these have detrimental effects on physical health, all three act as stimulants rather than relaxants so do little to help people relax properly. Drugs such as cannabis that are said to help people relax can act as a depressant and users can become paranoid and lose ambition and drive. Not only that, drug use and drinking alcohol can cause or exacerbate mental health problems.

There are many positive ways to relax that can have a better impact on your mental health. There are a few techniques that can prevent stress rising throughout the day.

⇨ Pausing – take time throughout the day to take a break or a pause. Stop what you are doing, look out of the window, let your shoulders drop, stretch and allow your mind to calm down. Taking several pauses throughout the day can prevent stress from building up. If you encounter a stressful situation such as an upsetting phone call, a busy train ride home, writing an essay, give yourself time afterwards to calm down.

⇨ Deep breaths – often people are told to 'take deep breaths' after a stressful situation and sometimes concentrating on your breathing helps the body to relax and can have a calming effect. To aid with this relaxation technique, close your eyes, take deep breaths in and out. Think of your favourite place, maybe somewhere that you like to go

on holiday. Focus on that and think about that place and what you might be doing there. You might remember sunbathing on a beach. You can smell sun tan lotion, you can hear the sea. Picturing this 'nice place' can help you to relax and take yourself away from the current stressful situation and help calm you down to prevent stress levels gradually rising throughout the day.

Top tips – ways to relax

⇨ Taking up a hobby – people who have stressful jobs often find that taking up a hobby can help them switch their brains off from work pressures once they are away from work. For example, if you are knitting, you are concentrating on what your fingers are doing rather than thinking about that essay that needs handing in next week that is stressing you out. Often when you go back to the thing that you were finding stressful, you can cope better having taken a break from it and switching off.

⇨ Aerobic exercise – exercise where the heart rate is increased releases endorphins which make you feel good. Exercises could include going to the gym or sport such as football or netball but could also include cycling, skate boarding, surfing,

riding a horse, swimming – think about the type of things you are interested in and build your exercise around that.

⇨ Walking – walking also releases endorphins but can also help you to switch off from pressures as you take in the scenery around you and get into a steady rhythm – and can be a far more pleasant way to travel than on a stuffy tube or busy loud bus which in itself can be stressful. Getting fresh air also helps you to relax and sleep better.

⇨ Yoga – yoga, tai chi and pilates are designed around relaxation and breathing techniques which can all aid relaxation.

⇨ A warm bath – it sounds simple but a nice warm bath helps the muscles relax and encourages a general feeling of relaxation. Aromatherapy candles or bubble bath could also help your mind to relax and some people find listening to chilled music while you are having a soak helps.

⇨ Watching a film or reading a book – escapism is a great way to switch off from reality for a while and help the mind to relax.

⇨ Meet a mate – leaving the stressful situation you are in and talking things over with a mate or even chatting about something completely different from what caused the stress can take your mind off things and aid relaxation.

⇨ The above information is reprinted with kind permission from YoungMinds. Please visit www.youngminds.org.uk for further information.

© YoungMinds 2013

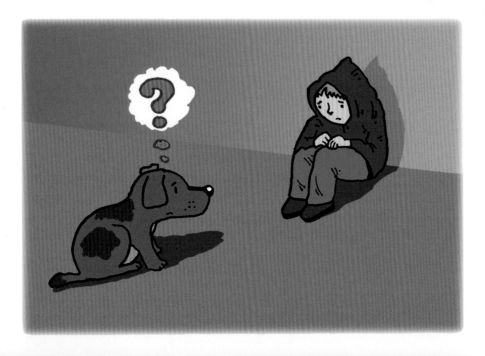

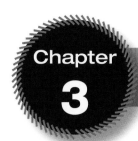

Teens worried over lack of sleep, according to the Schools Health Education Unit

Many teenagers do not believe they are getting enough sleep to remain alert at school and stay healthy, research suggests.

It reveals girls are more concerned about their sleeping habits than boys, and that youngsters are more likely to say they are not getting enough as they get older.

More than one in four 14- and 15-year-old girls (28%), and just over a fifth of boys of the same age (22%) do not think they sleep enough to concentrate on their studies, according to the Schools Health Education Unit.

Their findings, drawn from surveys of thousands of school children aged from ten to 15, show that fewer 12- and 13-year-olds (Year 8) are concerned about lack of sleep affecting their classwork.

A fifth (20%) of Year 8 girls, and 16% of boys said that the amount of sleep they normally get is not enough for them to stay alert and concentrate on lessons.

The research shows the proportions of youngsters who are concerned about the impact lack of sleep has on their health, with 17% of 12- and 13-year-old boys and the same number of girls saying they don't think get enough to stay healthy.

This rose to 22% among 14- and 15-year-old boys (Year 10) and 27% of girls of the same age.

Overall, 80% of Year 8 boys and 78% of Year 8 girls said that they get eight hours or more sleep a night, this fell 65% for Year 10 boys and girls.

The study also reveals that many youngsters are spending much more time playing the computer and watching TV than doing homework.

Asked how long they had spent doing homework the night before, 4% of 14- and 15-year-old boys said that they had spent more than three hours on it.

But almost a fifth (19%) of boys of this age said that they had spent more than three hours playing computer games, and 14% had spent more than three hours watching TV.

Among girls in the same age group, 10% had spent over three hours on homework, 5% had spent this long playing computer games, and 15% had spent over three hours watching TV.

Maggie Fisher, health visitor for parenting website Netmums said: 'Children, and teenagers in particular, are leading increasingly busy lives and we know this is leading to a sleep deficit. Research shows for each hour of sleep lost, IQ drops by a point so the cumulative effect of lots of late nights can have a serious impact on teenager's studies at school.

'Children nowadays spend far more time surfing the web or watching TV, so sleep experts advise all electronic devices to be switch of at least 30 minutes before bedtime or it can affect sleep quality and brainwave patterns.

'However, what we are seeing is many children sleeping with smartphones tucked under their pillows which prevents restful sleep.'

She added that teenagers have different sleep patterns to other people, making them more likely to go to bed later and get up later.

Mike Griffiths, vice president of the Association of School and College Leaders (ASCL) said: 'As this survey suggests, there's a general concern at the amount of time youngsters are spending interacting with screens, whether TV or computers, as opposed to interacting with people.'

Mr Griffiths suggested that lack of sleep could be linked to the amount of time spent playing computer games or watching TV.

He said he was not sure if taking part in these activities makes children more or less tired than going outside and playing a game like football.

But he added: 'Some of these videos and interactive games are not very restful. With physical activity perhaps you get a good night's sleep.'

Mr Griffiths said that in some cases, it may be that parents are telling a child to go to bed, saying goodnight and then a little later the child is back up playing computer games in their bedroom.

22 July 2012

⇨ The above information is reprinted with kind permission from the Press Association. Please visit www.pressassociation.com for further information.

Why are teens always tired?

Trouble getting up on school days, dozing off in class, marathon lie-ins at weekends ... You'd be forgiven for thinking teenagers sleep their lives away.

In fact, the opposite is true. Sleep experts say teens today are sleeping less than they ever have. This is a worry, as there's a link between sleep deprivation and accidents, obesity and cardiovascular disorders.

Physiological changes, social pressures and external factors such as TVs and other stimulating gadgets in the bedroom contribute to late nights and mood swings.

Lack of sleep also affects teenagers' education, as it can leave them too tired to concentrate in class and perform to their best ability in exams.

Teen sleep thieves

Our sleep patterns are dictated by light and hormones. When light dims in the evening, we produce a chemical called melatonin, which gives the body clock its cue, telling us it's time to sleep.

'The problem is that society has changed,' says Dr Paul Gringras, consultant paediatrician and director of the Evelina Paediatric Sleep Disorder Service at Guy's and St Thomas' Hospital in London.

'Artificial light has disrupted our sleep patterns. Bright room lighting, TVs, games consoles and PCs can all emit enough light to stop the natural production of melatonin.'

Other distractions include mobile phones and instant messaging, which teens may use well into the night.

These all worsen the usual changes taking place in the body during adolescence, which means teenagers fall asleep later in the evening.

'That wouldn't be a problem if there was no need to get up early in the morning for school,' says Dr Gringras.

'The early-morning wake-ups mean they're not getting the average eight to nine hours of sleep. The result is a tired and cranky teenager.'

Several school districts in the US have introduced later start times for pupils in an effort to improve their performance, although results have been mixed.

How the body clock affects sleep

'Catching up on sleep at weekends isn't ideal. Late nights and long lie-ins further disrupt the body clock,' says Dr Gringras.

In severe cases, an individual's body clock can be so different to everyone else's that they can't fall asleep until late at night. This condition is called delayed sleep phase syndrome (DSPS). It's similar to the feeling of jet lag and is a disorder of the body's timing system.

Treatment for DSPS includes bright light therapy – such as exposure to a bright light for about half an hour every morning – and chronotherapy, which involves restoring the individual's natural sleep phase.

'Sometimes we give a small dose of melatonin in the evening, about an hour or so before bedtime,' says Dr Gringras. 'Over the long term, this helps to reset the body clock.'

'However tired they feel, they should avoid lie-ins at the weekend. They should get exposure to outdoor light,' he says.

Getting help for sleep problems

A range of services for sleep problems can be accessed through the NHS. Your GP can tell you more about this.

Dr Gringras says: 'Your doctor will also be able to give you basic advice on addressing sleep issues and, where appropriate, recommend a sleep clinic.'

2 April 2013

⇨ The above information is reprinted with kind permission from NHS Choices. Please visit www. nhs.uk for further information.

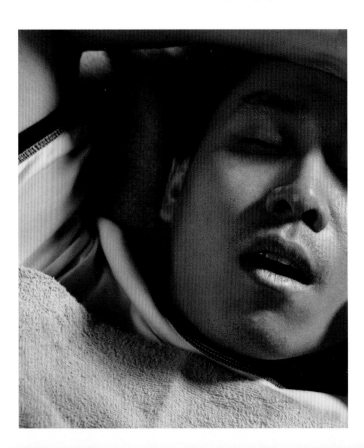

A nation raised on crisps and fizzy drinks?

The British Heart Foundation has carried out a survey of what secondary school children eat. It isn't, needless to say, a blameless diet – but nor is it quite as noxious as the BHF pretends.

By Nigel Hawkes

OnePoll, an organisation that uses online panels for carrying out surveys, gathered responses from 2,002 children aged 11 to 16 between 6 and 19 September this year. It asked first what the children normally ate for lunch, and got 6,743 responses – so, as you would expect, most respondents ticked more than one box.

A quarter said they had school dinner, and 61 per cent a sandwich (filling unspecified). Just over a fifth said a chocolate bar, almost a third fruit, just over a third crisps, 18 per cent yogurt, 8.6 per cent soup and 9.0 per cent salad. That doesn't sound very surprising, or especially dreadful. It isn't out of line with studies made of the contents of packed lunches by the School Food Trust, using a bigger sample and a much better methodology, but with primary rather than secondary school children.

The OnePoll survey also asked children what they drank. This attracted 3,947 responses so each respondent ticked, on average, two boxes. More than half said they drank water and 47 per cent squash, with more than a third saying fruit juice. Nearly a third said fizzy drinks, divided almost equally between diet and non-diet versions, and 7.4 per cent said energy drinks. But since there is an overlap it's impossible to conclude from this that a third drink nothing but fizzy drinks or indeed a third nothing but fruit juice.

More illuminating answers came from the question: 'On an average day, how many times do you eat chocolate, crisps or sweets?' The commonest answer, from 39 per cent of respondents, was once a day; 26.6 per cent said twice a day, with smaller numbers saying any number up to ten times a day.

The poll interprets this as an average of 2.19 times a day, but that is not the right measure. To avoid distortion by those claiming a huge intake of sweets or crisps, the median is better than the average. The median in this case is closer to one than two – it's about 1.25.

Where I take exception to the BHF is in its claim, drawn from the results of the survey, that a child's typical daily diet includes 'one packet of crisps, one chocolate bar, one bag of chewy jelly sweets, one fizzy drink and one energy drink'. From this it calculates children are consuming 118 g of sugar a day and more fat than a cheeseburger contains. The survey results cannot bear this interpretation.

The median child (or kid, as the BHF prefers) consumes 1.25 items a day that fall into the 'chocolate, crisps or sweets' category, yet the BHF claims the typical daily diet includes three items falling into this category. As for drinks, only 20.5 per cent of all responses listed fizzy and energy drinks. It is not reasonable to claim from these results that a typical child drinks one of each every day.

Needless to say, all the papers that reported the survey used the 'typical diet' claim, when the actual results suggest that such a diet would be completely untypical. That's not to say that children are eating a perfect diet, or even close to one: but they certainly aren't doing as badly as the charity seems to believe on the evidence of its survey.

I suspect the 'typical diet' claim was concocted to justify the BHF's headline: 'The real five-a-day? UK kids feast on chocolate, energy drinks and crisps'.

23 November 2011

⇨ The above information is reprinted with kind permission from Full Fact. Please visit www.fullfact.org for further information.

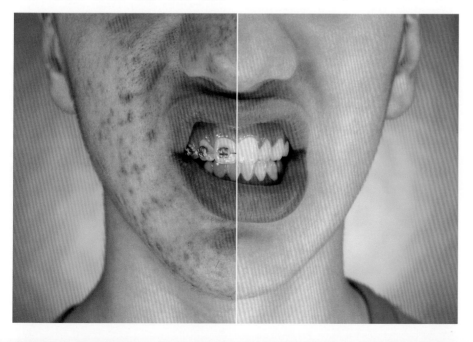

School food standards chip away at teens' unhealthy eating

Fewer teenagers are having chips for school lunch since legislation to improve school food came into full force, new research has found.

Our national study – the first of its kind in secondary schools since compulsory nutritional standards came into full effect in 2009 – shows that the proportion of young people on school meals who had chips for their lunch was down from 43% in 2004 to 7% in 2011.

It also shows that almost all schools had ditched the sale of chocolate, sweets and crisps completely since the introduction of the legislation (although almost three quarters of students having packed lunches were still bringing these types of foods into school), and that the average school meal being eaten by secondary school pupils contained around a third less saturated fat, fat, salt and sugar in 2011 than it did in 2004.

However, as the number of secondary school students having school meals continues to rise, the research also shows that schools still need to do even more to encourage them to fuel up well for their afternoon lessons.

Despite huge improvements to what's on the menu, teenagers are still not choosing food combinations that will give them enough energy and nutrients to stay alert all afternoon. Whilst the number of pupils having fruit, veg or salad with their lunch has doubled since the legislation came into force this still needs to increase much further, and teens are still not eating enough of their 'five-a-day' as part of their school meal.

We'll be outlining a series of recommendations arising from the findings in the coming weeks, after completing our research on the approaches to food being taken by academy schools.

Our senior nutritionist Jo Nicholas, who led the secondary school research, said: 'These findings show that even just 12 to 18 months after the final standards came into effect, as many secondary schools were getting to grips with the changes, the legislation was already making a significant impact – not just for what was on the menu but also for what teenagers were actually eating. Instead of 'chips with everything' we're starting to see signs of 'chips now and again'.

'It's also very clear that it's tougher for secondary schools to encourage students to make better choices than it is for primary schools, often because there are such a huge range of options on the menu. Caterers need to keep innovating to get teenagers eating even more fruit and veg, and to encourage them to have combinations of foods that will fuel them up properly.

'Ultimately, this research shows the really positive impact of the standards on the food on offer to young people at school, and on what they actually eat, in a short space of time.'

The study looked at:

⇨ Fruit and veg: schools still need to do more to get students eating fruit and veg. In 2004, only 59% of secondary schools had veg or salad on the menu every day. Now, almost all do (98%). The number of pupils taking a piece of fruit or a portion of veg or salad with their lunch has doubled since the standards were introduced, and almost three quarters of students now have at least some vegetables, pulses, fruit or fruit juice as part of their lunch – a sign that caterers are innovating to get fruit and vegetables into all sorts of dishes. However, the average number of portions being taken with lunch across all pupils was just 0.8 – and this must be improved.

⇨ Starchy foods cooked in fat or oil – like chips, Yorkshire puddings and garlic bread: more than three quarters of schools (77%) used to offer foods cooked in fat or oil every day – now it's just over half of schools that do this (53%). Now these sorts of foods are being served on around 3.5 days per week, down from 4.2 days per week. The standard says these foods should not be on offer more than three times per week, so the caterers are making real progress. Most importantly, fewer pupils are eating these foods – the percentage fell from 50% of pupils in 2004 to 17% in 2011.

⇨ Chips: the proportion of pupils having chips for their lunch was way down – now at 7% of pupils, compared with 43% of pupils in 2004. Also, chips were on the menu far less often – on 17% of days in 2011 compared with 80% of days in 2004 – and most chips were being cooked in healthier ways. Potatoes cooked in oil were on the menu on 59% of days in 2011 compared with 89% of days in 2004. This is much better, but still too often.

⇨ Sweets, chocolate and crisps have almost completely disappeared. In 2004, three quarters of schools offered confectionery and crisps every day as part of the lunch menu. Now, almost all schools have ditched them completely.

- Cereal bars: often just as high in sugar as confectionery, these are still being served when they shouldn't be on offer – something that needs to be made clearer to caterers.

- Pizza: in 2004, two-thirds of secondary schools used to offer pizza every day – that's now down to only half, and pupils are actually eating pizza less often.

- Water: in 2004, only three quarters of schools (68%) offered water as a drink at lunchtime – now almost all schools do (98%).

- Nutrient content: now, the average school meal is more packed with nutrients than it was in 2004. The average meal being eaten now contains around 50% more vitamin A, and around a third less saturated fatty acids, salt, sugar and total fat than it did in 2004.

It follows our findings on the impact of the standards in primary schools, published in 2010.

Our chairman, Rob Rees, said: 'Regulation may not always be popular, but evidence doesn't come much clearer of the difference it can make in tackling poor diet – one of the most serious and costly public health issues we face.

'If we want our schools to be places where children's minds and bodies are well-nourished, it's abundantly clear from this research that the standards should be the very minimum we expect for food in all schools.'

28 April 2012

- The above information is reprinted with kind permission from Children's Food Trust. Please visit www. childrensfoodtrust.org.uk for further information.

Survey suggests fewer teens are using illegal drugs

Teenagers across England appear to be leading a cleaner lifestyle.

A survey of 6,500 children aged 11-15 revealed that over the past decade the numbers taking drugs, smoking and drinking alcohol had all fallen.

Data from the NHS Health and Social Care Information Centre figures found 17% had tried drugs at least once in 2011, compared with 29% in 2001.

The survey is conducted every year to monitor use of drugs, alcohol and cigarettes and focuses on a selection of secondary school pupils, with the latest carried out between September and December.

It found that among 15-year-olds who had tried drugs, the number fell from 39% in 2001 to 23% in 2011 and the figure for children aged 11 was only 3%.

The number of teen smokers was the lowest since the survey began in 1982 with 5% saying they smoked at least one cigarette a week compared with 10% in 2001.

Those drinking alcohol at least once dropped to 45%, from 61% in 2001.

Tim Straughan, chief executive of the NHS Health and Social Care Information Centre, said: 'The report shows that pupils appear to be leading an increasingly clean-living lifestyle and are less likely to take drugs as well as cigarettes and alcohol.

'All this material will be of immense interest to those who work with young people and aim to steer them towards a healthier way of life.'

The charity Drinkaware said the report was good news but warned there were still 360,000 young people who reported drinking alcohol in the last week alone.

27 July 2012

- The above information is reprinted with kind permission from Healthcare Today. Please visit www.healthcare-today. co.uk for further information.

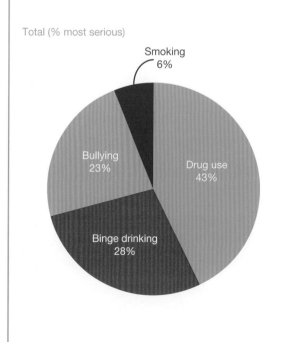

Plese rank the following issues in order of how serious you think they are for young people (under-18s) today?

Total (% most serious)

Smoking 6%

Bullying 23%

Drug use 43%

Binge drinking 28%

Source: Populus Limited, Phillip Morris International Survey of public attitudes on tobacco packaging, July 2012, London.

43 deaths linked to legal highs

More than 40 deaths were linked to a group of now-banned legal highs in 2010, eight times as many as the previous year, figures have shown.

By Wesley Johnson.

The biggest increase related to meow meow, which rose from five deaths in 2009 to 29 the following year, the National Programme on Substance Abuse Deaths report showed.

Methcathinones, which include meow meow and have since been made class B drugs, 'tightened their grip on the recreational drug scene in western Europe but especially the British Isles', the report said.

It went on: 'The rapidity with which these new substances have emerged appears to be at an increasing rate.

'In the past, the market for new psychoactive substances to explore evolved steadily over much longer periods of time.

'It is now difficult to gauge with any certainty what will be the next "big thing" that will capture the attention of the experimenter or regular recreational drug user.'

Deaths from use of methcathinones – which include mephedrone, commonly known as meow meow – rose to 43 in 2010 from five the previous year, the figures based on information from coroners showed.

Controls on previous legal highs such as ketamine, piperazines, and so-called date-rape drugs GHB and GBL helped reduce their popularity, the report said.

Overall, drug-related deaths in the UK fell by almost 14% to 1,883 in 2010 from 2,182 the previous year.

Professor Hamid Ghodse, director of the International Centre for Drug Policy (ICDP) at St George's Hospital, London, which released the report, warned against complacency.

'There are indications that there is still a general upward trend in fatalities involving emerging drugs such as mephedrone and prescription drugs such as methadone,' he said.

'This is a great concern and it is clear that much work is still required in improving access to effective treatment and rehabilitation services, and, most importantly, finding prevention strategies to stop people being at risk in the first place.'

A Department of Health spokeswoman said: 'Any death related to misuse of drugs is a tragedy for the victim, their families and their friends.

'So-called legal highs are not a safer alternative to illegal drugs. As with any substances, the risks increase if you combine them with alcohol or other drugs.'

She went on: 'Our drugs strategy aims to get people off drugs and stay off drugs and from next year, local authorities will be given a ring-fenced public health budget to tackle local public health issues.

'This will offer real opportunities to integrate drug treatment and other local services.'

The number of drug-related deaths in England fell to 1,358 from 1,524 in 2009, while in Scotland the number of deaths fell to 365 from 479, and in Wales they were down to 81 from 102.

In Northern Ireland, the number of drug-related deaths rose to 72 from 65, the figure showed.

In the UK, around three-quarters of deaths were of men (1,386) and three in five were aged 25-44 (1,135).

The highest rate of drug-related deaths per 100,000 population aged 16 and over in 2010 was in Brighton and Hove (14.8), followed by Manchester (13.4), Blackpool and The Fylde (11.8), Fife (10.3), and Lothian and Borders (10).

7 November 2012

⇨ The above information is reprinted with kind permission from *The Independent*. Please visit www.independent.co.uk for further information.

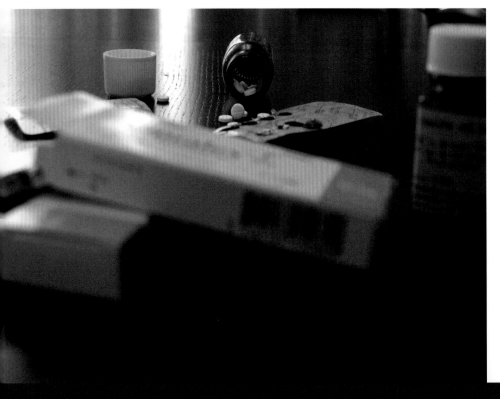

Students taking 'smart drugs' Modafinil and Ritalin may lead to drugs testing around exam time

Students could face compulsory drugs testing around exam time amid concerns that some are 'cheating' by taking pills to improve their results.

Research show 10% of UK students admit to taking 'cognitive enhancing' drugs to help them concentrate, stay up late and complete deadlines on time. This rises to 16% among US students.

Professor Barbara Sahakian, a psychiatrist at Cambridge University, told *The Independent*: 'People are starting to think about drug testing. Some of the students who don't use cognitive enhancers may demand it because they are concerned about cheating. Some admissions tutors are also concerned about it.'

Ritalin, usually prescribed for attention deficit disorder, and Modafinil, prescribed for narcolepsy, are some of the most favoured 'performance enhancers' named by the report of a joint Academies workshop into Human Enhancement and the Future of Work, published online on Wednesday.

These drugs are being chosen by students and academics alike because they 'do not produce extreme changes in mood that usually accompany recreational use, such as a "high" or "rush", and do not lead to obvious physical dependence' the report says.

However, Professor Sahakian pointed out research into the long-term effects of taking such drugs had not been explored.

The report also explored how use of 'cognitive enhancing' drugs had reached the workplace. Professor Sahakian said: 'The head of one laboratory in the US said that all of his staff are on modafinil and that in the future there will be a clear division between those who use modafinil and those who don't.'

A 2011 study found that modafinil reduces impulsive behaviour and improves cognitive flexibility in sleep-deprived doctors. Unlike caffeine, which in higher doses is accompanied by tremor and heart palpitations, this is not seen with modafinil.

However, neuroscientist Jack K. Lewis, blogged on Huffington Post UK about the dangers of believing the promise of such 'wonder' drugs in November, saying one study 'highlighted the gap between people's expectations and the actual effects of such substances'.

'In sleep-deprived individuals a single dose of modafinil does have a strong positive effect on executive function and improvement in memory – an effect that wears off during continued sleep deprivation.

'But were they to take a single dose when not sleep deprived, they would find it has the opposite effect – under these conditions it actually induces drowsiness. Furthermore, repeated doses of modafinil when not sleep deprived increases both positive and negative affect, which means you would simultaneously feel slightly happier and more anxious.

'My message to school kids (or their parents for that matter) who might be considering buying into the promise of Ritalin-enhanced grades? Don't believe the hype.'

There are serious ethical implications of enhancements like these being necessary for jobs or degrees. In the Introduction the report states: 'Enhancement could benefit employee efficiency and even work–life balance, but there is a risk that it will be seen as a solution to increasingly challenging working conditions, which could have implications for employee well-being.'

Jackie Leach Scully, an ethicist at Newcastle University, told *The Guardian*: 'We've worked very hard in this country and elsewhere to put in place legal requirements to have tolerable working conditions and the last thing we'd want to see happening is for that to slip away.'

The *Human enhancement and the future of work* report also explored how technology such as bionic arms could be used as physical enhancements in the workplace.

7 November 2012

⇨ The above information is reprinted with kind permission from *The Huffington Post*. Please visit www.huffingtonpost.co.uk for further information.

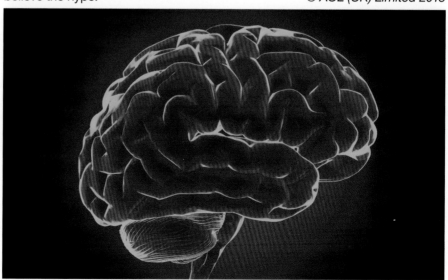

Smart drugs: would you try them?

Having seen the effect drugs like Modafinil have had on my friends, I'm steering clear.

By Tom Newman

Have you ever wondered what it would be like to have access to instant genius in the form of a little pill? In the run-up to last summer's exams, curiosity proved too great a temptation for a few of my mates. They got their hands on a substantial haul of Modafinil, a prescription-only drug normally used to treat narcolepsy.

Modafinil is one of a number of performance-enhancing smart drugs that can be found online. It gives a sensation of natural wakefulness for hours at a time, without the jittery buzz and disrupted sleep associated with caffeine.

It also sharpens the mind, boosts memory and aids problem-solving: the Ministry of Defence shipped thousands of pills to tired soldiers in Afghanistan and Iraq.

They certainly work. While I was dozing off, bored senseless by revision, my mates were more focused than a Buddhist monk mid-meditation.

But modafinil does more than just keep you awake. I asked a friend who tried it out to describe his experience.

'It messes with your mental reward system,' he said. 'It makes you desperate to do what you know you actually need to do. You just don't want to do anything else. I wanted to revise all the time, non-stop.'

Professor Barbara Sahakian, a leading neuroscientist at the University of Cambridge, explained it to me in scientific terms: 'Our recent study published in *Neuropharmacology* suggests that healthy people use smart drugs, like modafinil, to get down to and complete tasks that they have been putting off, because these tasks seem more enjoyable when taking these drugs.'

In short, drugs like modafinil make revision seem fun. This might sound like everything a stressed student could want, but prospective pill-poppers should be warned – the pills come with a whole range of potential physical side-effects.

'At present there are no long-term safety studies of these drugs in healthy people,' explains Professor Sahakian. 'We know that the brain is in development into late adolescence. Therefore we do not know the long-term consequences of the effects of these drugs on a healthy developing brain.'

Ordering online, she adds, is 'a very dangerous way to obtain prescription-only drugs. You do not know what you're actually purchasing.'

In my experience, modafinil changes people's behaviour too. Over those weeks my friends became different people – in turn aggressive, cold and reclusive. Eating was 'a waste of time' and so was conversation.

One friend, a world-class procrastinator, could be found swearing at anybody who interrupted his work flow, walking away from conversations mid-sentence. When I put it to another that using brain-enhancing drugs amounted to cheating, he turned on me, accusing me of wanting to ban revision. He apologised the next day. He said it was the drugs talking.

It's easy to see the appeal of modafinil. It's readily available on the Internet – a month's supply would set you back around $50, apparently – and unlike that other popular study drug, Ritalin, possession without prescription isn't actually illegal.

A spokesperson for the charity DrugScope says Modafinil is a prescription-only medication but not a controlled substance, so it is not illegal to be caught in possession of it. However, under the Medicines Act, it is an offence to supply, which includes everything from wholesale dealing to simply giving some to a friend.

Ritalin, however, is a controlled substance under the Misuse of Drugs Act, the spokesperson says. Possession of it without a prescription is illegal and it is a Class B drug.

A BBC survey found that of those people who had tried smart drugs before, 92% would do so again. My friends say they'd happily do so, maintaining that they're not put off by the health risks.

Nor do they consider smart drugs a form of cheating, comparing the practice to paying for tutoring or private schooling.

I'll admit that I was intrigued – but not enough to try it. Having seen the bizarre behaviour of other users, I find the effects unsettling and, frankly, a little bit scary.

Modafinil may promise to change your grades, but it might also change the way you act. Don't say you haven't been warned.

24 October 2012

⇨ The above information is reprinted with kind permission from *The Guardian*. Please visit www. guardian.co.uk for further information.

The Hermione Granger effect: why teenagers are finally starting to say no to drugs and alcohol

Report shows that pupils appear to be leading an increasingly clean-living lifestyle.

By Jeremy Laurance

Say goodbye to the drug-fuelled raver and hello to the clean-living ecowarrior. Teenagers are changing and, for perhaps the first time in history, their parents approve.

'Among 11- to 15-year-olds, the proportion who admitted to having taken drugs fell from 29 per cent in 2001 to 17 per cent in 2011'

Rates of drug-taking, drinking and smoking among children have plummeted in the past decade. Girls, it seems, are more likely to emulate the polite, studious Hermione Granger, played by Emma Watson in the Harry Potter films, than wild-child party girls like Peaches Geldof in her heyday.

Among 11- to 15-year-olds, the proportion who admitted to having taken drugs fell from 29 per cent in 2001 to 17 per cent in 2011. Regular smokers of at least one cigarette a week halved from one in ten to one in 20. The number who said they had drunk alcohol in the past week was down from 26 per cent to 12 per cent.

Experts said a 'profound shift' had taken place in the new generation's attitude to drink and drugs. The findings were based on a survey of 6,500 children aged 11 to 15 at secondary schools in England, conducted between September and December 2011.

Tim Straughan, the chief executive of the NHS Health and Social Care Information Centre, said: 'The report shows pupils appear to be leading an increasingly clean-living lifestyle and are less likely to take drugs as well as cigarettes and alcohol. All of this material will be of immense interest to those who work with young people and aim to steer them towards a healthier way of life.'

Siobhan McCann, of the charity Drinkaware, said: 'While the decline in the number of children trying alcohol is good news, the report still shows there are 360,000 young people who reported drinking alcohol in the past week alone.

'Parents are the biggest suppliers of alcohol to young people aged ten to 17 and also the biggest influence on their child's relationship with drink.'

Drug-taking, drinking and smoking increases with age, the study found. Among 11-year-olds, fewer than one in 30 said they had taken drugs in the past year, compared with almost one in four 15-year-olds.

Cannabis was the most popular drug but its use fell during the decade. In 2011, one in 13 young people said they had smoked it, compared with one in seven in 2001.

Drug use was found to be highest in southern England and lower in the Midlands and the North. The proportion of children saying they had smoked cigarettes at least once was the lowest since the survey was first carried out in 1982 – reflecting the pressure created by anti-smoking laws. Even so, one in five said they had tried cigarettes and one in 20 did so regularly.

In 2001, one in five teenagers said they drank alcohol at least once a week. By 2011, that proportion was down to one in 14. Miles Beale, of the Wine and Spirit Trade Association, said: 'The increase in the number of young people who have never drunk alcohol, and the fact those who do drink appear to be drinking less, suggests that the messages about the risks of underage consumption are being heard.'

'Most of us think of our future, and drink won't help'

Rosie Brighton, 13, Watford

'I know a few people my age that drink but not many. When you look at people that turn up for school hung-over, not caring and not getting the grades, it is off-putting. Most of us are working hard to get good exam results because we look at the high unemployment rates and think we'll need all the help we can get. We're thinking about our future,

'Most of us think of our future and drink won't help'

and drink is not going to help that.

'I don't know anyone who smokes or takes drugs. A lot of people are afraid of how mad their parents would be if they were caught. I think health authorities and schools have to educate children about drugs early. I had my first lesson in school about drugs in Year 6, but have been made aware of the dangers by my mum.'

27 July 2012

⇨ The above information is reprinted with kind permission from *The Independent*. Please visit www.independent.co.uk for further information.

© independent.co.uk 2013

Binge drinking: more than just a student problem

By Helen Charman

The emergence of a study conducted by the HealthyFit group at the University of Vigo shows that female students binge drink more than their male counterparts by a significant percentage, echoing a study published in 2010 by the London School of Economics detailing the fact that more educated women are likely to be heavier drinkers: this isn't just a phase to be consigned to student days, like taking too many photographs and wearing knitwear in bed to save on heating.

The inevitable hand-wringing from prominent responsible adults about the recklessness of the youth of today, throwing around the phrase 'Skins-generation' with all the cultural ease of David Cameron's repeated bizarre hymns to Angry Birds, is sure to kick off soon, but rather than tread these tired paths of displaced responsibility, the productive thing to do is to ask why this happens. We all know how bad binge drinking is for you, and a night out in any university town is far more effective than any Drink Aware campaign in displaying both the popularity and the undeniably explosive (So classy! So cost-effective!) effects of binge

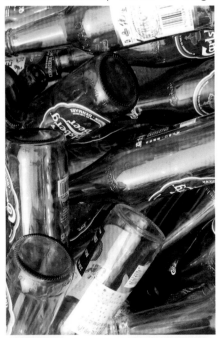

drinking, yet downing half a bottle of vodka three nights a week is a far from abnormal student experience.

This isn't an example of an unusual deviance within our generation, a predilection for booze that has sprung out of nowhere: if you want to know why students are drinking so much, look to the context we've grown up with, the behaviours we've learned. In my first week at university I was told by a senior member of staff that the institution 'runs on alcohol', that it lubricates everything that occurs in the place: we've grown up in a society that uses alcohol consumption, in no mean quantity, as a mark of adulthood, of sophistication, a liquefied symbol of coming of age. The quality of the alcohol consumed may differ – swapping Sainsbury's house Soave for Tawny Port – but the behavioural patterns there are the same.

Of course there are social pressures involved – of drinking societies, of Freshers' Week bonding, of sports team initiations – and of course it our own peer groups who perpetuate these, but excessive alcohol consumption, at a safe distance, over a fry up the next morning or laughter at amusing stories from the night before, is often treated by even the most responsible of the responsible adults we know as an endearing trait that is the mark of a normal, socially active student, the benign evidence of high-spirited youth and a fulfilled university experience. Talking to your parents about that smoking habit you've happened to pick up or the joint you roll occasionally would be met, nine times out of ten, with horror or at the very least disapproval, but drinking a bottle of wine in one sitting is nothing out of the ordinary: after all, it's a wholesome family activity when done over Christmas dinner.

Compared to previous generations, those of us currently at university are quite spectacularly unfortunate: fee rises, the poor housing market

and graduate unemployment are all conspiring to create a perpetually gloomy outlook which has contributed to the rise of a 'f*** it' culture, the ubiquity of the almost unbearably witty phrase 'YOLO' suggesting that if we're graduating into a world of debt, stress and competition anyway, we might as well enjoy ourselves while we can.

This could also offer an explanation as to why binge drinking is demonstrably more of a female than a male problem, despite the stereotype of rugby lads drinking until they prove they are in fact medical marvels constructed entirely from testosterone: the Future Foundation think tank released research in 2012 detailing the particular pressures put upon young women in our society, suggesting we are actively preventing young women from fulfilling their potential by focusing on weight, on looks and sex appeal, destroying self-confidence and self-worth and all the other good things beginning with self, perhaps creating a need to escape into the oblivion drink can offer, or creating a greater need to use alcohol as a social crutch.

So if you're looking for reasons why students are drinking such terrifying amounts, and why female students are in particular, look not for signs of abnormally addictive personalities, or bad behaviour, or a lack of concern for health in our generation: look to the examples and pressures provided by the society that has been created for us. It's enough to make anyone reach for a double, or a bottle.

3 January 2013

⇨ The above information is reprinted with kind permission from *The Huffington Post* UK. Please visit www.huffingtonpost.co.uk for further information.

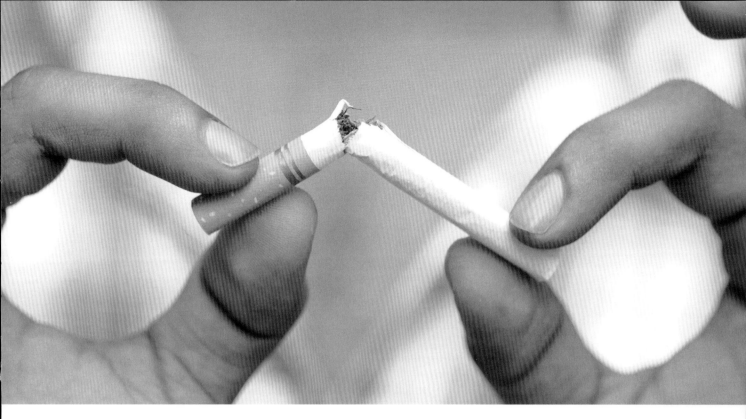

Young people and smoking

Smoking prevalence

It is estimated that every year more than 200,000 children in the UK start smoking.[1] Among adult smokers, about two-thirds report that they took up smoking before the age of 18 and over 80% before the age of 20.[2] The latest survey of adult smokers shows that almost two-fifths (39%) had started smoking regularly before the age of 16.[3]

The annual government survey of smoking among secondary school pupils in England defines regular smoking as smoking at least one cigarette a week. However, in 2011 pupils classified as regular smokers smoked a mean (average) of 35.6 cigarettes a week, approximately five a day. Occasional smokers consumed on average 3.5 cigarettes a week.[4] The number of cigarettes smoked by both regular and occasional smokers has fallen significantly since 2007.

The proportion of children who have ever smoked continues to decline. In 2011, 25% of 11- to 15-year-olds had smoked at least once, the lowest proportion since the survey began in 1982 when 53% had tried smoking.[4] Previously, girls had been more likely than boys to have ever smoked and to be regular smokers. However, in 2011, a similar proportion of boys and girls said they had tried smoking (25% and 26%, respectively). The

prevalence of regular smoking increases with age, from less than 0.5% of 11-year-olds to 11% of 15-year-olds.[4]

The decline in smoking has been most marked among older pupils. The proportion of 14-year-olds who smoked regularly fell from 13% in 2006 to 7% in 2011; among 15-year-olds, 11% smoked regularly in 2011, compared with 20% in 2006.[4]

What factors influence children to start smoking?

Smoking initiation is associated with a wide range of risk factors including: parental and sibling smoking, the ease of obtaining cigarettes, smoking by friends and peer group members, socio-economic status, exposure to tobacco marketing, and depictions of smoking in films, television and other media.[5]

Children who live with parents or siblings who smoke are up to three times more likely to become smokers themselves than children of non-smoking households.[6] It is estimated that, each year, at least 23,000 young people in England and Wales start smoking by the age of 15 as a result of exposure to smoking in the home.[5]

Smoking, alcohol and drug use

There is a strong association between smoking and other substance use. The 2011 secondary school survey found that of the 8% of pupils reporting that they

1 *Childhood smokers*. Cancer Research UK, March 2013

2 Robinson S and Bugler C. *Smoking and drinking among adults*, 2008. General Lifestyle Survey 2008. ONS, 2010.

3 Office for National Statistics. *General lifestyle survey overview: A report on the 2010 general lifestyle survey*. 2012.

4 *Smoking drinking and drug use among young people in England in 2011*. The Information Centre for Health and Social Care, 2012'

5 *Passive smoking and children*. Royal College of Physicians, London, 2010 (pdf).

6 Leonardi-Bee J, Jere ML and Britton J. *Exposure to parental and sibling smoking and the risk of smoking uptake in childhood and adolsecence: a systematic review and metaanalysis.* Thorax 15 Feb 2011 doi:10.1136/thx.2010.153379.

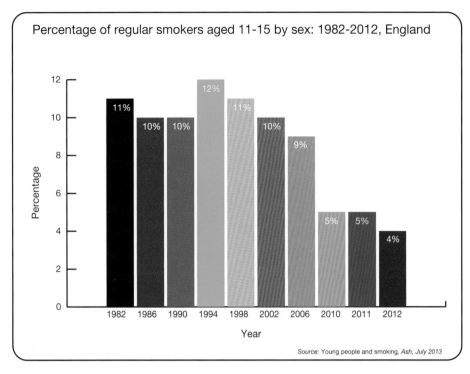

Percentage of regular smokers aged 11-15 by sex: 1982-2012, England

Source: Young people and smoking, Ash, July 2013

and persist in the habit as adults, the greater the risk of developing lung cancer or heart disease.[8]

Children are also more susceptible to the effects of passive smoking. Parental smoking is the main determinant of exposure in non-smoking children. Although levels of exposure in the home have declined in the UK in recent years, children living in the poorest households have the highest levels of exposure as measured by cotinine, a marker for nicotine.[9]

Bronchitis, pneumonia, asthma and sudden infant death syndrome (cot death) are significantly more common in infants and children who have one or two smoking parents. For more information see the ASH Research Report: *Passive smoking: the impact on children*, ASH Factsheets: *Smoking in the Home, and Smoking in cars*.

had smoked cigarettes in the week prior to the survey, the majority (5%) had also drunk alcohol or taken drugs recently, or both.[4]

Other factors associated with smoking

Young people who played truant from school or who had been excluded from school in the previous 12 months were almost three times more likely to smoke regularly compared to those who had never been truant or excluded.[4]

Attitudes to smoking

The proportion of pupils who think it is acceptable to try smoking has decreased since the question was first asked in 1999. Currently, 35% believe it is acceptable to try smoking to see what it is like. compared with more than half in 1999. Children's views of what they believe is acceptable for someone of their age tends to reflect actual behaviour with slightly more believing it is OK to try smoking (35%) compared to those who actually do so (25%).[4]

Smoking and children's health

The younger the age of uptake of smoking, the greater the harm is likely to be because early uptake is associated with subsequent heavier smoking, higher levels of dependency, a lower chance of quitting, and higher mortality.[5]

Child and adolescent smoking causes serious risks to respiratory health both in the short and long term. Children who smoke are two to six times more susceptible to coughs and increased phlegm, wheeziness and shortness of breath than those who do not smoke.[7] Smoking impairs lung growth and initiates premature lung function decline which may lead to an increased risk of chronic obstructive lung disease later in life. The earlier children become regular smokers

Addiction

Children who experiment with cigarettes can quickly become addicted to the nicotine in tobacco. Children may show signs of addiction within four weeks of starting to smoke and before they commence daily smoking.[10] One US study found that smoking just one cigarette in early childhood doubled the chance of a teenager becoming a regular smoker by the age of 17[11] and a London study suggests that smoking a single cigarette is a risk indicator for children to become regular smokers up to three years later.[12] In the 2010 survey of schoolchildren in England, 67% of regular smokers reported that they would find it difficult not to smoke for a week while 73% thought they would find it difficult to give up altogether.[13] During periods of abstinence, young people experience withdrawal symptoms similar to the kind experienced by adult smokers.[14]

Smoking prevention

8 BMA Board of Science. *Breaking the cycle of children's exposure to tobacco smoke*. British Medical Association, London, 2007.

9 *Going smoke-free. The medical case for clean air in the home, at work and in public places. A report on passive smoking by the Tobacco Advisory Group of the Royal College of Physicians*. London, Royal College of Physicians, 2005.

10 Di Franza JR et al. *Initial symptoms of nicotine addiction in adolescents*. Tobacco Control 2000; 9: 313-319.

11 Jackson C and Dickinson D. *Cigarette consumption during childhood and persistence of smoking through adolescence*. Arch Pediatr Adolesc Med. 2004; 158: 1050-1056.

12 Fidler JA et al. *Vulnerability to smoking after trying a single cigarette can lie dormant for three years or more*. Tobacco control 2006; 15: 205-209.

13 *Smoking, drinking and drug use among young people in England in 2010* The Information Centre for Health and Social Care, 2011.

14 McNeill AD et al. *Cigarette withdrawal symptoms in adolescent smokers*. Psychopharmacology 1986; 90: 533-536.

7 *Smoking and the Young*. Royal College of Physicians, 1992.

Research suggests that knowledge about smoking is a necessary component of anti-smoking campaigns but by itself does not affect smoking rates. It may, however, result in a postponement of initiation.[15]

High prices can deter children from smoking, since young people do not possess a large disposable income: studies suggest young people may be up to three to four times more price sensitive than adults.[16] In Canada, when cigarette prices were raised dramatically in the 1980s and the early 1990s, youth consumption of tobacco plummeted by 60%.[17]

An American study has shown that while price does not appear to affect initial experimentation of smoking, it is an important tool in reducing youth smoking once the habit has become established.[18] The National Institute for Health and Clinical Excellence (NICE) has issued guidance on school-based interventions to prevent the uptake of smoking among children.[19]

Children, smoking and the law

On 1 October 2007 the legal age for the purchase of tobacco in England and Wales was raised from 16 to 18. The amendment was designed to make it more difficult for teenagers to obtain cigarettes, since, despite the law, children still succeeded in buying tobacco from shops and vending machines. In 2008, the first time data were collected after the change in the law, 39% of pupils who smoked said they found it difficult to buy cigarettes from shops, an increase of 15% from 24% in 2006.[20] There has also been a drop in the proportion of regular smokers who usually buy their cigarettes from a shop: from 78% in 2006 to 58% in 2010.[13] The 2010 survey also found that 8% of 11-15-year-old regular smokers reported that vending machines were their usual source of cigarettes, compared to 17% in 2006.

A ban on the sale of cigarettes from vending machines entered into force in England on 1 October 2011. A ban on the display of tobacco products in retail outlets is being introduced in two stages: from April 2012 in large shops such as supermarkets and in April 2015 in small shops.[21]

During 2009 there were 216 prosecutions in England and Wales for underage tobacco sales, with 175

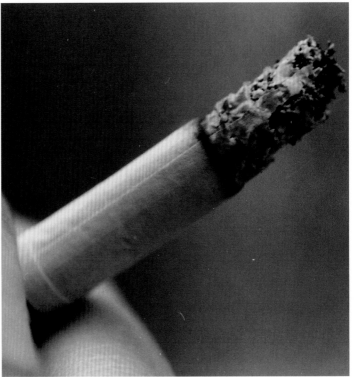

defendants being found guilty.[22] An amendment to the Criminal Justice and Immigration Act includes banning orders for retailers who persistently sell tobacco to persons under the age of 18. These measures came into force in April 2009.

Legislation alone is not sufficient to prevent tobacco sales to minors. Both enforcement and community policies may improve compliance by retailers but the impact on underage smoking prevalence using these approaches alone may still be small.[23] Successful efforts to limit underage access to tobacco require a combination of approaches that tackle the problem comprehensively.

March 2013

The latest smoking, drinking and drugs surgey is available at http://hscic.gov.uk/catalogue/PUB11334.

⇨ The above information is reprinted with kind permission from ASH: Action on Smoking and Health. Please visit www.ash.org.uk for further information.

15 Reid D. et. al. *Reducing the prevalence of smoking in youth in Western countries: an international review.* Tobacco Control 1995; 4 (3): 266-277 (pdf).

16 Hopkins, D et al *Reviews of evidence regarding interventions to reduce tobacco use and exposure to environmental tobacco smoke.* Am J Prev Med 2001; 20: 16-66.

17 Sweanor D and Martial LR. *The Smuggling of tobacco products: Lessons from Canada.* (Non-Smokers Rights Association, 1994).

18 Emery S. White M and Pierce J. *Does cigarette price influence adolescent experimentation?* J Health Economics 2001; 20: 261-270.

19 *School-based interventions to prevent the uptake of smoking among children.* NICE, March 2010.

20 *Smoking, drinking and drug use among young people in England in 2008.* The Information Centre for Health and Social Care, 2009.

21 Health Act 2009.

22 *Offences relating to the illegal sale of tobacco to underage persons – England and Wales, 2003 to 2009.* Office for Criminal Justice Reform, 2011.

23 Lancaster T and Stead LF *Interventions for preventing tobacco sales to minors.* The Cochrane Library, Issue 4, 1999

⇨ Mortality rates amongst young people aged 15-19 and 20-24 have risen above rates for those in the one to four age group, a reversal of historical mortality trends. (page 1)

⇨ In 2010 the under-18 conception rate had fallen again, to 35.5 per 1,000 girls aged 15-17, down from 47.1 in 1998, and the lowest rate for decades. (page 1)

⇨ There are 7.6 million young people aged ten to 19 in the UK, making up 12% of the population. (page 3)

⇨ Teen cancer is the leading cause of non-accidental death in young people in the UK. Over 2,500 young people aged 13-24 years are diagnosed each year. (page 3)

⇨ One third of those aged 11-15 in the UK are overweight, one in six obese. Less than half meet minimum exercise requirements. (page 3)

⇨ 29% of young people in England aged 15 have experimented with illegal drugs at some point and 28% are drinking regularly, which impacts on crime levels, accidents and A&E admissions. (page 3)

⇨ A school-age child will see their GP on average between two and three times per year. (page 4)

⇨ Under half of respondents said they got most of their health information from a health clinic, and just under half said they would talk to their GP if they were worried about their health. (page 5)

⇨ Only 14% of respondents to the National Children's Bureau survey said they had not felt stressed in the previous week. The most commonly cited sources of stress were school work or exams, concerns about their future career, and their physical appearance. (page 5)

⇨ One in ten five- to 16-year-olds in the UK have a clinically diagnosable mental health problem. (page 6)

⇨ Around 1.1 million children and young people (one in 11) in the UK have asthma, making it the most common long-term medical condition. (page 7)

⇨ Around one in 500 children in the UK develop some form of cancer by the age of 14, making it the most common cause of death from disease for children and young people. (page 7)

⇨ Type 2 diabetes is now being diagnosed more frequently in younger overweight people and is most prevalent among children and young people of South Asian origin. (page 8)

⇨ Some 600,000 people in the UK have epilepsy – around 1% of the population – with young people under 18 accounting for around 10% of this total. (page 8)

⇨ In the *Understanding Society* survey from the ISER, staying out late without parents' knowledge was reported by 21% of boys and 15% of girls aged ten to 15. It was more common in boys and older children (page 12)

⇨ A recent study has suggested that 15% of young people have an episode of anxiety at some point. (page 13)

⇨ Around one in 100 children are affected by depression before they reach puberty and three in every 100 teenagers are affected. Depression is twice as common in girls than in boys. (page 18)

⇨ Recent research from Ohio State University Medical Center shows that late-night exposure to light from a television or computer screen could be a risk factor for depression. (page 20)

⇨ One in ten young people (ten per cent) feel they cannot cope with day-to-day life, warns a new report from The Prince's Trust. (page 21)

⇨ The Prince's Trust Youth Index reveals, based on interviews with 2,136 16 to 25-year-olds, shows how more than one in five young people (22 per cent) did not have someone to talk to about their problems while they were growing up. (page 21)

⇨ Most young people who harm themselves are aged between 11 and 25. The age at which most people start is 12, but some children as young as seven have been known to do it. (page 22)

⇨ A study, headed by scientists from the University of Las Palmas de Gran Canaria and the University of Granada, found that fast food consumers, compared to those who eat little or none, are 51% more likely to develop depression. (page 24)

⇨ More than one in four 14- and 15-year-old girls (28%), and just over a fifth of boys of the same age (22%) do not think they sleep enough to concentrate on their studies, according to the Schools Health Education Unit. (page 27)

⇨ Research show 10% of UK students admit to taking 'cognitive enhancing' drugs to help them concentrate, stay up late and complete deadlines on time. This rises to 16% among US students. (page 33)

⇨ Among 11- to 15-year-olds, the proportion who admitted to having taken drugs fell from 29% in 2001 to 17% in 2011. Regular smokers of at least one cigarette a week halved from one in ten to one in 20. The number who said they had drunk alcohol in the past week was down from 26% to 12%. (page 35)

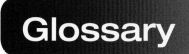

Adolescent

A young person - someone in a transitional phase between child and adult.

Anxiety

A feeling of nervousness or worry.

Binge Drinking

Consuming a large volume of alcohol in a short period of time, often with the intention of becoming intoxicated.

Cardiovascular Disorders / Disease

Problems that affect the heart and circulation.

Cognitive Enhancer

A substance that improves mental functions such as memory, recall and concentration.

Depression

A feeling of low mood which can affect a person's behaviour, feelings and thoughts.

Exam Stress

A feeling of nervousness, fear or worry before or during a test.

Legal High

Drugs which are intoxicating but not illegal.

Long-Term Condition

A medical condition that cannot be cured but can be eased or controlled with medication.

Mental Health

The state of a person's psychological well-being.

Methodology

The methods or systems used to undertake research or an area of study.

Nutritional Standards

A set of regulations set by the government to ensure that the food served in schools provides a healthy, balanced diet for children

Psychoactive Drug

A drug that affects the brain function; often resulting in changes of mood, behaviour or perception-levels.

Recreational Drug

A drug that is taken occasionally and is often claimed to be nonaddictive.

Risky Behaviour

Behaviour that has the potential to get out of control or become dangerous.

Self-Harm

An intentional harming of one's own body.

Stereotype

A fixed idea of a certain type of person or thing.

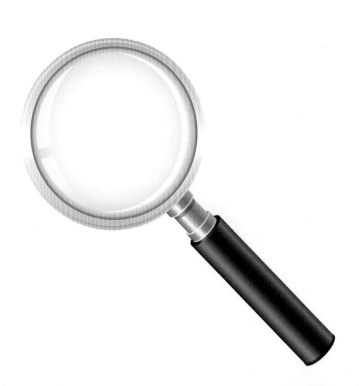

Assignments

1. Interview your parents, teachers or others who are older than you and find out how healthy they were when they were younger. How much exercise did they do? What were their diets like? Do they feel healthier now? Write some notes and feedback to your class.

2. Teenage conceptions, cigarette smoking and cannabis use amongst teenagers have all declined since 2008. However, rates of obesity and sexually transmitted infections have both increased. Choose one of these trends and plan a campaign that will help to tackle its rise amongst adolescents in the UK. Your campaign could take the form of television ads, web banners, posters on buses… whatever you think would be most effective and accessible to the target age-group. Your plan should include samples and a mission statement detailing your goals and how you intend to achieve them.

3. Diagnoses of long-term conditions such as diabetes, epilepsy and asthma are increasing amongst young people in the UK. Research one of these conditions and create an information booklet for parents that will help them to spot warning signs. You could also include information on where they can go for support.

4. Read the article *Ten reasons for investing in young people's health* on page 3 and choose one of the ten reasons listed. Write a letter to your local MP using your chosen reason to emphasise the importance of investing time and money in teenage health.

5. In pairs construct a questionnaire that will be distributed throughout your school/college to investigate young people's opinions on their local health services. Write a report that summarises your findings. Include graphs and tables to illustrate.

6. Write a blog entry exploring why teenagers are more likely to indulge in risk-taking behaviour than other age groups – for example, smoking, drinking alcohol and using illegal drugs.

7. In small groups discuss the dangers of young people staying out late without telling their parents where they are or what they are doing. Do you think it is necessary for teenagers to inform their parents where they will be?

8. With a partner, list the things that can make young people anxious and try to think of some coping mechanisms.

9. Design an app that will give students tips and advise on how to cope with exam stress.

10. Write an article for your local newspaper exploring the issue of depression amongst young people.

11. Create an advice booklet explaining the issue of self-harm. Include suggestions of where teenagers can go for help and support.

12. Research alternative treatments for depression such as healthy diet, increased exercise and herbal remedies. Create a sample 'healthy body, healthy mind' plan for teenagers aged 14- to 16-years-old. Consider the types of food and activities that would appeal to this age-group. For example, you could include recipes, meal-plans or exercise ideas and create a booklet that will be handed out at your local schools.

13. Write an article exploring why sleep is important for adolescents.

14. 'Taking "smart drugs" to boost exam performance is totally harmless.' As a class, debate this motion.

15. Watch the 2011 film *Limitless*, starring Bradley Cooper. In the film Bradley Cooper's character takes a pill that allows him to access 100 per cent of his brain's abilities. Write a review exploring the positive and negative effects this pill and consider what message the Director was trying to convey to his audience. (Note: Limitless is rated 15 and contains some scenes of violence).

16. What are the dangers associated with binge-drinking? Create a poster that demonstrates your ideas.

17. Do you think the new laws regulating cigarette packaging and displays have helped to reduce the amount of teenagers who smoke? Discuss with a partner.

Acknowledgements

While every care has been taken to trace and acknowledge copyright, the publisher tenders its apology for any accidental infringement or where copyright has proved untraceable.

Illustrations:

Pages 5 & 22: Don Hatcher; pages 7 & 22; Angelo Madrid; pages 3 & 20: Simon Kneebone.

Images:

All images are sourced from iStock, Morguefile or SXC, except where specifically acknowledged otherwise.

Pages 9 & 32: Jackie Staines.

Additional acknowledgements:

Editorial on behalf of Independence Educational Publishers by Cara Acred.

With thanks to the Independence team: Mary Chapman, Sandra Dennis, Christina Hughes, Jackie Staines and Jan Sunderland.

Cara Acred

Cambridge

September 2013